The Pathway Home

A Guide to Divine Inner Healing

By

Peter Monroy M.D.
Elizabeth Monroy M.S.

Published by Infinite Human Productions (second edition)

www.infinitehuman.com

Text copyright © 1996 by Peter Monroy and Elizabeth Monroy Printed in U.S.A.

First Edition printed at Montana Litho & Bindery, Sun River, Montana

Second Edition

The information in this book was originally published in 1996 under our publishing House: Going Home Books over twenty-five years ago. Obviously much has changed in our world and our current global healthcare system in the past twenty-five years. While I have updated much of the information I have sought to persevere the original integrity of my husband's work for two reasons: One: To demonstrate that much of what we warned about over twenty- five years ago has come to pass and now defines today the delivery of "modern" medicine. And two: To demonstrate how if something is not corrected it will spread and bleed into every aspect of our lives as we have now observed with the advent of our Global Heath Care Crisis. We have seen how the Americanized modal of Modern Medicine has become the basic principles used by the W.H.O. (World Health Organization) to dictate the Draconian Mandates that have been issued in every country around the World as the only way to cure C.O.V.I.D.

No Part of this book may be reproduced or transmitted by any means, electronic or mechanical, including photocopying, recording or by information storage and retrieval system, except by a reviewer who may quote brief pas sages in a review to be printed in a magazine or newspaper—without permission in writing from the publisher.

For more information contact:

www.infinitehuman.com or infinitehumanproductions@gmail.com

DISCLAIMER

The data contained in this book is based upon information from intuitive knowledge, published sources and directly from spiritual teachers. The authors make no warranties, expressed or implied, regarding the complete ness of this information, nor do they warrant the fitness of the information for any particular purpose. This information is not intended for use in connection with the sale of any product. This summary of information from intuitive knowledge, books, medical articles and other sources is not intended to replace the advice or attention of health care professionals, or replace their independent professional judgement. If you have any problem with your health, contact a health care professional for advice. The names of any individuals' are used fictitiously. Any resemblance to persons, living or dead, is entirely coincidental.

Library of Congress Card Catalog Number 96-75268

ISBN: 978-1-958184-17-2

Second Edition published by Infinite Human Productions Published by GOING HOME BOOKS

Cover design by Paul Amit

Edited by Toni Chavez, Gay Whiteside and Sandra Hatzfeld.

Final edit by Marsha Covington.

Text design and formatting by Michael Dougherty.

ACKNOWLEDGEMENTS

Our deepest appreciation to Toni Chavez whose input during the early stages of this book was priceless. Our thanks to Gay Whiteside, for her honest review of a later draft and to Sandra Hatzfeld, whose gentle touch transcended, the book to a higher level. Finally, our eternal gratitude to all our teachers, both seen and unseen.

DEDICATION

To Sharon and Patrick.

FOREWORD

When I (Peter), was five years old growing up in Cuba, I had my first extraordinary experience that everyone in my family was quick to dismiss as a hallucination. Sometime after going to bed, a glowing open hand appeared at the window and moved close to my bed. At first I was frightened by the apparition, but gradually I realized it meant me no harm. I continued to stare at it until it disappeared. Years later I read a book that referred to a similar event as the hand of God calling a soul to service.

My next extraordinary experience occurred when I was an adult living in New England. Every night I saw myself lift out of my physical body and go through walls. I also heard the sounds of bells and people talking, although I was completely alone. At first, I was convinced I was having a nervous break down and decided not to tell any one. Some time passed until information concerning this event came to me as I read a book on astral travel in which the author related an experience identical to the one that I had.

As my life unfolded, I observed that there seemed to be two duplicate worlds: one of societal perception and the other a world of expansive enormity on whose threshold I stood. It seemed as if I were being drawn into this other world and, if I allowed myself to go with the flow, interesting things would always ensue.

It was in this manner that I met Elizabeth, my wife, ten years ago. I had just arrived in Florida and she was there for a few days, on her way to California. It was a chance encounter on a beach where we were brought together by the sight of a dead shark. I now realize the Universe was communicating to me through the symbol of a dead fish representing the death of my own spirituality. This was indeed the state Elizabeth found me in. Until then I had still been seeking spiritual answers within the confines of organized religion. I had even begun to doubt the existence of God because I could not reconcile my extraordinary experiences with the information I was being given by my religious teachers.

Elizabeth was much different from anyone I had ever met. She had a strong dedication to God, yet, understood the limitations of organized religion. According to her, anything was possible through the individual's own connection with God. We argued constantly over spiritual matters, my lack of faith and everything under the sun. How could two people be so different, yet be so much in love? Despite our arguments, we both knew at some level we had been together many lifetimes and had reunited to make the final journey Home. Charged with a higher purpose, we embarked on our spiritual journey and began the task of blending our energies. A year later we decided to take a sabbatical and felt compelled to visit my relatives in the Canary Islands of

Spain. During our twomonth stay we resided in an old cave house that had been in my family for over three hundred years.

Our days were simple, spent mostly reading, meditating and exploring the islands. It was during one of those meditations that I was spiritually awakened by a tremendous vibrating wave which started in my groin area and traveled slowly to the top of my scalp. The force of this energy was so great I panicked, thinking I would surely die. As the wave moved up my body with penetrating force, I realized something wonderful was occurring and allowed myself to relax. When the experience was over, I rushed to tell my wife. With great excitement I recounted the incredible event. Elizabeth told me it was a spontaneous rising of the Kundalini. From that day on I knew there was much more to me than what I had learned in my religious upbringing or my formal education.

A few months later we picked up a spiritual book and in it found the phrase, "When the student is ready the teacher will appear." We remember wondering if it was all that simple "Ask and you shall receive!" So for the next few months we concentrated all our efforts on asking the Universe to provide us with a teacher, one who would guide us to the highest spiritual level possible. Over the next six years we read literally hundreds of books ranging from self help and Eastern philosophies to the Kabala and magic. The more we read, the more we realized how little we both knew. Until one day, when we least expected it, we were directed toward our teachers. Through this memorable relationship came a wealth of knowledge and wisdom that forever changed our lives. Our meeting made the purpose of writing this book clearer. The book would serve as a foundation for correct thinking, correct action and living in accordance with God's Will in a time of great need. The book would also prepare individuals to bring more Light into their bodies. As you read the next two hundred plus pages, do your best to rid yourself from old judgements and allow the written symbols to speak to your soul.

Table of Contents

Section One: The New Healer — 1
   1. Physician Heal Thyself — 2

Section Two: The Four Natures — 14
   2. Physical Wellness — 15
   3. Emotional Wellness — 24
   4. Mental Wellness — 32
   5. Spiritual Wellness — 40

Section Three: Dis- Ease and Modern Healthcare — 50
   6. Dis- ease — 51
   7. The Global Health Care Crisis — 57

Section Four: Social and Financial Evolvement — 72
   8. Greed (in America) — 73
   9. Government and Power — 79
   10. Organized Religion — 87

Section Five: The Four Human Activities — 98
   11. Relationships — 99
   12. Work, Education, Playtime, and Devotion — 109

Section Six: The Pathway Home — 123
   13. Self Responsibility and Doors — 124
   14. Home — 136

Section One:

The New Healer

*An evolved healer
is the first step in restoring
Spiritual wellness to a dis- eased society.*

CHAPTER 1
PHYSICIAN HEAL THYSELF

About twenty-five centuries ago a man named Hippocrates founded what is known today as modern medicine. He believed that to become a physician required not only knowledge and skills but a life long commitment to help others without harming self or others in the process. *Prim um non nocere* (First do not harm). He also taught his students that to achieve wellness, a healer must treat the whole patient and not just the dis- ease. Hippocrates also found that the environment in which the patient lived greatly effected the type of illness and its severity. The lifestyle, diet and stress level a patient experienced commonly dictated what illness would be manifested in the individual.

It seems ironical that, in the modern world of medicine, many methods that Hippocrates, the father of modern medicine, employed would be considered "alternative medicine." Oddly enough, what is now known as traditional or allopathic medicine is a recent byproduct of the medical sciences, whereas nontraditional medicine, such as energy work, herbology and homeopathic remedies, have been around much longer. Perhaps it is time we switch names, since historically speaking, modern medicine is the new kid on the block.

The Healing Arts have evolved into two distinctly separate camps: traditional and non traditional medicine. As politics dictate, these two groups are constantly trying to discredit and negate the others accomplishments and usefulness. Why not instead merge traditional and non traditional medicine and evolve the Healing Arts to a higher level? As new healers emerge from the blending of these two sciences, the Healing Arts will be in a unique position to evolve beyond the Hippocratic teachings using the vehicle of science to bring spirituality into the physical form.

Through the integration of these two contributing branches, this new breed of healers will treat not only the physical body, but also the emotional, mental and spiritual bodies to achieve true wellness. In this fashion medicine can evolve into a union between patient and healer as they work together to achieve a common goal. The patient accepting responsibility for his/her dis- eased state thus works as a cohealer with the physician/healer. By utilizing the best from both worlds, providers can offer a broader array of options for their patients.

In Ancient times the role of a healer was also that of a holy man, or spiritual leader. The healers job was to see where spirit was blocked in the afflicted and how to best assist the person in becoming unblocked, allowing spirit to flow through them with ease, unhindered. These medicine men, Shamans or spiritual leaders role was mystic in nature. They possessed the ability to "see" into the various spiritual levels and dimensions to perform work there. The Shaman, or holy man studied all aspects of the human and spiritual realms to determine how to return the individual to wholeness. This advanced mode of healing brought the spiritual and the physical worlds together. This a very sacred activity and only the most evolved souls were permitted to engage in it. To the Native Americans someone who had powerful medicine possessed a strong connection to the spiritual world. These souls had to themselves be whole (Holy).

It is interesting to look at what motivates most individuals to become healers. I (Peter), know in my own case, I've often looked back at the choices I made and what influences precipitated my decision to apply to medical school and specialize in obstetrics and gynecology. Beginning with my own birth process, I can now identify a few dramatic events that played a role in making that decision. I was born in a small town in Cuba in the 1940s and arrived four weeks late by cesarean. At that time having surgery frequently led to post operative complications and even death. In my mothers case the infection that set in after my birth led to a pelvic abscess that required a hysterectomy with removal of both ovaries when she was thirty-two years old. In those days estrogen was not routinely given to young women who were surgically thrown into menopause, often crippling these unfortunate souls to a life plagued with emotional problems. Years later my father discussed this devastating event with me and cried as he said, "Your mother and I never had sexual relations after that ordeal." At some level I believe I had been punishing myself for all the pain and suffering I caused my mother at birth. However, with increased awareness I now realize there are no accidents and everything is preplanned with our counselors before the birth process. My mother knew at some level that this was a karmic debt that she had to pay.

Perhaps because of this bond, she and I developed a close relationship that lasted well into my adulthood years. This tight relationship also effected my decision to become a doctor, because my mother later worked professionally as a nurse/midwife. I also believe there was something deeper—a call to serve humanity through the Art of Healing—that I could not ignore. What is even more incredible is the journey I took to become a healer.

My interest in becoming a doctor began as a teenager while I was finishing high school through Adult Basic Education evening classes. The reason I completed my high school education at night was due to my fleeing Cuba when Castro came to power, prior to completing my secondary education. I arrived in Miami at age sixteen, penniless, alone and unable to speak English. After integrating into the culture of this country, I began taking my studies seriously. I continued to work days while I finished college with an engineering degree. Soon after graduating from a small New England college, I realized becoming an engineer was not satisfying my life's purpose, so I decided to apply to medical school. My decision to further my schooling came as a surprise to my family and friends who felt that becoming an engineer was impressive enough. To the amazement of myself and others, I beat the forty to one odds and gained acceptance into an internationally famous medical school in Boston. All my energies went into the pursuit of becoming a doctor. My insatiable desire to join a profession filled with tradition, responsibility, power and awe at the understanding of the human body negated every other aspect of my life. As I submerged myself into my professional career, time ceased to exist. I recall spending endless nights selfabsorbed in my studies. Why was I so driven? Was my life destined from the beginning to answer the propelling call with in me to heal?

I now realize that there had been something in me all along which drove me to the limits of human endurance and caused my detachment from human relationships. My innate knowledge (carried from one lifetime to the next) and my pursuit of new knowledge was obviously of greater importance to my souls complete unfoldment than anything else. Physicians have a gift or talent similar to that of painters, sculptors, writers, singers, teachers or cooks. It is the gift to assist others in their healing through the artistic expression of their skill. By using their intuitive awareness they may reach a deeper understanding of the human condition. A good physician combines skill with intuition. A great physician has two additional attributes: compassion and love. A true healer has such great compassion that s/he radiates love at such a powerful level people can be healed simply by being in their presence. Christ and other Ascended Masters are living proof of this phenomenon. Being a healer is rewarding in so many ways that it is hard to explain the exchange that takes place between the physician and the patient. One of the greatest joys of my life has come from the simplicity of a patient's smile and in knowing that we have both evolved during the healing process. So it is puzzling to me that so many of my colleagues are unhappy in their professional and/or personal lives. Why is my profession so laden with alcohol and drug abuse? Why is the incidence of divorce, depression and burn out among the highest in the medical profession?

Physicians, as all healers, subconsciously bring their personal unresolved issues into the healing arena. Because counseling programs are not included as an integral component of physician training, these individuals come to accept that they are beyond emotional entanglements. They are groomed to be "gods." The system teaches doctors emotional detachment not only from patients, but also from themselves. Healers have forgotten that to properly practice their art they must first become whole within themselves. They have forgot the link between the past traditions of the Healing Arts and modern high-tech medical training.

In the ancient days of Hippocrates, perfect health was achieved when the afflicted were assisted in restoring balance to the four principal bodily fluids (cardinal humors). These humors were blood, phlegm, choler (yellow bile) and melancholy (black bile). Health and temperament of the body depended on the proportion of each fluid circulating at any given time. By relating these various bodily fluids to the emotional states of the individual's lifestyle and environment, a cure was often achieved. The healer was considered a counselor and a teacher who appreciated that a successful treatment depended on consideration of the whole individual, his/ her environment and lifestyle. This is how holistic medicine was born!

As the distance between humankind and Mother Earth grew over the centuries, modern medicine evolved into a science that compartmentalized the human body. Physicians and patients alike have lost the capacity to appreciate the existence of anything beyond a specific physical affliction. Regard for the individual as a whole being has become all but extinct in allopathic medicine. Modern Western medical science has dissected the essence of the human condition to fluid, bone and soft tissue. This dissected perspective separates physicians from the awareness that a whole life comes to them to be healed.

The physical body is only one of the "bodies" you house. Modern medicine limits its focus to the physical body and within this small circumference it has been subdivided into specialties, forcing doctors to limit their practices to specific body parts. Physicians have become high-tech mechanics, servicers and replacers of body parts and system analyzers without the awareness of the complexity of the entire system.

Physicians are placed in an impossible demigod position by their educators and colleagues. In addition, patients generally view them as perfect, believing their medical judgements are the only true choices available to them. If all around they are seen as icons, how can doctors admit they are not Godlike?

Adding to the stress is the belief held by many physicians that because they are godlike, they are not likely to err as other humans are. This inflated role is taught throughout the making of a doctor. The profession often attracts individuals with very large egos, who thrive on the rush of power they get from holding a life in their hands. At one level a physician needs to have a high level of confidence when operating in life or death situations, however, this double edged sword can also be very taxing on the physician. This powerful sensation is only transitory.

The first time a physician experiences a patient's refusal to cooperate in his/her own healing or that something has seriously gone wrong, the power dissipates. This is precisely why it behooves physicians to remember that they are not solely responsible for an individual's care. They are cofacilitators with the patient as the patient enters into his/her own healing. During my early clinical years in medical school, I recall observing and examining patients with obvious overtones of illness or depression only to have lab tests contradict what my senses had observed. Even the chief resident would say to me, "Well, Peter, as you can see all the lab results are negative, therefore Mrs. Jones's problem is clearly suprtentorial (in the mind)." So the modern day physician stops with the lab results. Can you imagine? We stopped where we should have started.

Over the centuries progress in the medical sciences has been measured according to how much understanding physicians have at a cellular level regarding how a specific illness occurs. Presumably we arrive at a cure for a dis- ease like cancer when we understand at the molecular level exactly what biochemical step goes wrong. With cancer, the oncologist, or cancer specialist, bombards cells that are rapidly dividing with chemotherapy. This treatment kills the "good" and the "bad" cells. Similarly, the surgeon cuts out the cancerous tissue in hopes that the patient's own immunological system (body defenses) will prevent a recurrence of the tumor. Unfortunately, none of the life patterns that led to the initial cancer have changed in the patient and the cancer returns, often with a greater force.

This Western mode of treatment by physicians negates any sense of responsibility the patient may have concerning his/her own illness. When a life pattern is not addressed by the physician or the patient, a door is left wide open for the recurrence or spread of a dis- ease. Until physicians recognize that a patient's belief system is directly connected to his/her dis- ease, only one aspect of the dis- ease will continue to be treated. A person's thoughts are directly connected to their physiology. A good example of this intricate connection is what happens when you've been embarrassed and your cheeks flush almost immediately. Thought patterns enter the body and either assist the body in directing the energy of the body in a balanced manner or they lock up the body and dis- ease strikes. The patient holds certain thought patterns which direct energy in the form of informational patterns throughout the body. These are electrochemical impulses which are transmitted to specific areas in the body causing physical reactions proportional and according to the individual's belief systems.

So what does all of this have to do with the wounded healer syndrome plaguing the modern day physician? Everything. Allopathic physicians have totally eliminated the patient's responsibility for maintaining good health and addressing the whole person instead of the dis- eased body part. Physicians have taken on the weight of total responsibility for the care and cure of their patients. Without this understanding of a healer/cohealer partnership, burnout will occur. Largely, because of this misperception many physicians are now suffering from battle fatigue. They have taken on a non ending battle against dis- ease, blinded by the erroneous assumption that the physical body is all that needs to be treated to achieve wellness and they are solely responsible for their patient's health. Just as soldiers, who know they are fighting a losing battle attempt to numb or escape their reality with mood altering drugs, so do many physicians retreat to their substance abuse trenches. It is therefore no wonder why many of my colleagues have given up on the medical profession altogether or chosen to take up the road of chemical dependency to deal with the daily stresses of their work.

It is usually at this burnout point that many physicians also recognize their economic trap, but continue to practice medicine despite the increasing dis- ease in other parts of their daily lives. Monetarily they have created a high profile lifestyle. I have a close friend, also an obstetrician, who exemplifies this scenario.

John has a private practice which incurs the expenses of medical malpractice insurance, an office mortgage, staff salaries, medical supplies, professional fees, and a professional community image. Personal expenses such as home mortgages, car payments, children's education and credit card payments keep John trapped in his current style of practice. Dealing with his burnout becomes a low priority for him since he must keep up with his expensive lifestyle. In an attempt to keep up with monetary standards, John orders more tests, schedules more surgeries, increases his patient load and creates even more stress. He works harder and longer hours until the stress level is so high he begins to ease it with a drink or two. He buys expensive toys to distract himself from his surmounting problems, which only add to his financial burden. He continues to play this role in an exclusive circle of high profile professionals, where each member tries to out do his/ her peer with external evidence of success. Thus, the "show and tell" game assumes the center stage as the competition cycle becomes a way of life. John builds a bigger house, buys a more expensive car, and lavishes his family with material *carte blanche* just to show everyone how great he's doing. He buys his way through the professional burnout. Now that he's got it all he's really happy, right?

For physicians to break out of this mold they must first admit something is not working in their lives. They then can begin to look for alternatives and options, not only in their own lives but in the ways in which they deal with the patients who seek guidance and assistance from them. The cycle perpetuates itself until the healer, John in this case, makes a conscious choice to heal himself.

Admittedly this personal momentous decision to shift from a high-powered lifestyle to simplicity is made with a great deal of courage, faith and detachment. The healer must shift his/her perspective back to the basics of the Hippocratic Oath: To assist humans with all skill and knowledge and without intent of harm in the practice of healing. This new perspective changes the very way in which s/he offers the practice of medicine. The new focus is on the evolving role s/he plays in his/her partnership with patients. This focus creates new opportunities, new possibilities. The old pattern of how s/he practiced medicine evolves from a material focus, interlaced with all the Medicare/Medicaid/private insurance systems, to a cleaner aproach of service as a physician/facilitator/healer.

Following the rule that one will attract to oneself what one needs to experience, a physician who needs to play the role of rescuer instead of facilitator will soon find a patient who needs rescuing. In the role of a rescuer, however, the physician may not see the appropriate treatment. The rescuer would want to rescue, but the facilitator would want to meet the highest need of the patient. Often patients (for reasons known only to themselves) will use an illness at a particular point in their lives to serve a greater purpose. The physician must be on the alert for those patients so that s/he may address his/her own needs to avoid playing the rescuer, manipulating the patient's illness in order to fulfill his/her personal power needs. Rescuers end up victims. By comparison, a facilitator would assist the patient in addressing the real issue behind the illness, discussing whether or not treatment was appropriate at the time. In these cases the physician will need to utilize intuition and medical knowledge to create an atmosphere evoking trust and cooperation. This openness in dialogue removes the physician from superiority to one of equal footing with the patient, thereby passing the ultimate responsibility of wellness onto the patient's shoulders. Few, if any, practitioners dare to use their intuition as a viable tool in the art of practicing medicine. My own training demanded that I deny it.

I am reminded of my experience with my former Chief of Service during my specialty training. He would not only discourage the use of intuition by his residents, but go to the extent of embarrassing them publicly when this approach was mingled with "sound medical advice." This man typifies the training most physicians receive today, which negates the existence of Divine Guidance which originates as a "gut feeling" available within them. Is it any wonder that physicians even recognize the spiritual essence of the human condition, their own or their patients?

As you have probably seen first hand, most healing practices work to negate the spiritual essence through the argument that the physical realm has properties which can only be seen, manipulated, probed and therefore able to be studied, understood, fixed or cured if dis- eased. Since Divine Intervention cannot be seen or measured by current scientific devices thus modern day physicians are unable to document this factor in the physical world. In other words, because they cannot quantify and subcategorize Divine Intervention into a doubleblind, crossover scientific study as they are used to, they omit it completely. They choose to follow standard medical procedures instead of allowing intuition and inner awareness to indicate that other factors may be present. An example of how incorrect this belief system is can be illustrated by my own personal experience with a former female patient.

Not long ago I was doing a hysterectomy on this patient who had three previous gynecological surgical procedures prior to coming to my office. Because of daily bleeding and pain during intercourse, we both decided a hysterectomy was the best solution to her problem. I was trying to save her from major surgery by doing a laparoscopy, which is surgery through a telescope inserted at the navel. The first thing I noticed was a lot of scar tissue. I felt a sudden chill go up my spine and with in a few moments my assistant slipped and fell to the floor. In thirteen years of private practice I have never seen that happen in an operating room. Instinctively I knew that I had received a sign—something had gone wrong with the surgery. I stopped the procedure and began to inspect more closely the operating field. A few moments passed and I found the answer to the sign. The end of the telescope had perforated the patient's large intestine! We immediately opened the abdomen and repaired the injury. Before we were finished, the bladder had to be repaired as well. Fortunately, the patient did well after the surgery without any complications or permanent damage. If this "accident" had gone unnoticed, the patient might have died.

I tell this story to illustrate the need for all physicians to be cognizant of other aspects of the patient. This requires time and greater insight into all four natures of the human being which obviously include the spiritual aspect as well.

Every day physicians, like everyone else, are presented with signs that tell them how they are doing on a professional and personal level. The trick is to pay attention to these signs and act on them accordingly. (This subject is discussed in chapter thirteen).

I have a close friend and colleague who recently went through a divorce which left him in financial ruin. The last time we spoke with one another he said to me, "Peter, I feel so angry. Damn it if I'm going to be a slave to my exwife." Soon after that he "accidentally" broke his wrist and could not operate for weeks. Have you ever had a situation where you can remember being the programmer of your brain and having something happen to you soon afterward? Can you see how powerful your thoughts are in directing energy to manifest dis- ease? Self injury? Healing? No matter what the final out come may be, energy will flow in the direction of your thoughts. If anger is the ruling force, as in the case of my friend, the outcome will most likely cause you harm in one form or another. To avoid this personal trap one must attend to all four natures. As stated in the beginning of this chapter, these four natures which all humans possess are: physical, mental, emotional and spiritual. It is crucial to remember to evolve a balance of all four aspects of these natures in every activity you undertake. These four human aspects must be addressed within every healing program undertaken.

Physicians also needs to listen to their own inner voices which will help them to help others. This is not the voice of the ego but instead a voice that speaks gently from the heart, a loving accepting voice that guides them through their daily lives. This is the voice of the higher self. For physicians this is one of their greatest tools both personally and professionally. Doctors can be great healers!

But the Healing Arts should not be confined to individuals with the letters M.D. or D.O. behind their names. As I (Peter), stated before, I felt a call to become a healer. My intuition told me that joining the Healing Arts was part of my purpose. Many of you may also feel this call leading you to work in different modalities. Many nontraditional healers today work in a variety of ways incorporating energy work, massage therapy, chiropractics, acupuncture, Ayurvedic principles, herbology and a variety of counseling services, just to name a few. It is important to remember that whatever form of the Art you use for healing, you must first seek wholeness within yourself. Then wellness will come to the patient seeking wholeness with you. By integrating all four natures into your treatment protocol, whatever modality you use, you will be of service in this time of great need.

As healers evolve and grow through the Art of Healing they must be aware of karmic repercussions which can occur within the Healing Arts. These individuals must be very careful in their practices not to accrue karma from their patients. This means they must be extremely clean with their healing work. By clean we mean they must be clear about their own issues which need to be dealt with and what their true role as a healer with a particular patient or client is. They must constantly strive towards their own wholeness, learning and evolving from each soul they have drawn to them, but not taking on their dis- ease. I always suggest to those on a healing path to find out why they are functioning within the Healing Arts. Once you know why you are doing it, evolve what you do to its highest spiritual level.

This may take the form of blending aspects of nontraditional and traditional methods and/or discovering your own unique style or signature within the Healing Arts. Once you have accomplished this goal, leave the HealingArts and move onto the next mode of self discovery. You must not get stuck doing the same thing over and over or you will accrue more karma. For example, our present role as "healers" has evolved into that of teachers. The word doctor comes from the Latin *doctres* meaning teacher and so presently we teach souls who are drawn to us a foundation so they can heal themselves.

As the energy focus shifts in the healer, so will it shift in the type of patients the healer attracts. Through this shift of belief systems, the physician and the patient draw into a kind of partnership. This partnership is based in the cooperative practice of medicine. Because like attracts like, the physician will begin attracting patients with whom s/he can practice his/her new philosophies. The patient's ability, conscious will, self responsibility and healing energy can bring about a cooperation that will allow the healing to take place.

As such healers hang their shingles, they will also discover they are growing and learning from the patients they attract. As physicians set aside their egos and come to the realization that the souls sitting across from them have a message for them also, they can enjoy and grow from the act of healing. For the most part, healers are not trained to listen to their patients and hear the real message. By really paying attention and seeing a soul, not a dis- ease, sitting across from them, a true healing can take place.

This holistic approach to allopathic medicine may take on the nature of consultation, physical examination, counseling, nutritional therapy, discussion with other members of the patient's family or an agreement to adjust the patient's current lifestyle. If the patient is a heavy smoker, or consumes a large amount of animal flesh, or lives a sedentary life—lifestyle changes can be suggested to shift the nature of risk factors in preventing dis- ease. If a patient has a more immediate risk factor such as a cardiac condition involving a dysfunctional valve, the physician can refer the patient to a heart surgeon to take care of the immediate medical need. After a successful operation, the initial caretaker can follow up with preventive lifestyle changes for the total success of wellness to the patient, or can make a referral to someone who can. Permanent lifestyle changes for a patient need to include the cooperation of immediate family members. Because the family is another "housing body" for the patient, all environments need to be treated in the recovery or prevention of dis- ease. Reaching that goal of wellness today may cost a high price in time, energy and dedication. But many individuals like ourselves, feel the time has come for medicine to evolve to a new level. This new level will allow physicians to incorporate all aspects of the patient's four natures, mental, physical, emotional and spiritual, during their treatment.

Many physicians will immediately dismiss these drastic changes in their practice because they may appear radical, impossible and/or impractical in the successful business of running a medical office. How a physician approaches the treatment of patients directly affects the monetary and time constraints of his/her practice.

According to current treatment standards, physicians have to see a certain number of patients each day to meet current monetary demands. It is unfortunate that many individuals enter the practice of medicine simply because it is viewed as an opportunity to make a lucrative living. Karmically, many physicians are digging themselves into a hole by placing the emphasis on the business aspect of medicine rather than on the Art of Healing and being of service. Additionally, Third Party Payers compensate physicians according to the quantity of care they produce rather than the quality, which emphasizes the incorrect practice of modern medicine. In my own case I (Peter), remember moving West expecting to set up another private practice and being concerned about meeting monthly expenses. As the opportunities presented themselves along my path, my worries never materialized, since I found myself working for a salary instead of the usual fee-for-service. This financial arrangement freed me to practice the purest form of medicine I had ever known. By combining a simple lifestyle with a salaried position I could meet all my financial obligations and have plenty of time for play. This also afforded me the opportunity to promote self responsibility on the part of the patient.

Ridicule may come from the idea of treating the patient as a co-healer. To eliminate the current standard role model of the God/doctor/healer with a cooperative/ facilitator, will not be viewed by many physicians as a positive move toward elevating the practice of medicine. But think how freeing it will be for physicians and patients alike. Responsibility will be taken off the shoulders of the healers and placed back where it belongs—on the shoulders of the patients. Doctors and individual patients do have the power to change the practice and the course of modem medicine. As the system exists today, both physicians and patients suffer the consequences and Karma of medicine's inadequate ability to meet the needs of both.

On a daily basis, physicians witness the mysterious power that gives life and takes it away, heals or disables. Why do physicians witness this power that is in all things but fail to recognize the connection that this power plays in providing monetary means in their own lives? This same miraculous, reparative power can provide for all your needs.

For those of you who are not healers it is important in today's world, as medicine becomes more controlled and regarded as a commodity, to learn to heal yourself, or at least start by fulfilling your role as a co-healer. This requires a greater degree of self responsibility and awareness. Our current bureaucratic system perpetuates the separation of body, mind, and spirit through its licensing laws where the doctors handle only the body, the counselors treat only the mind, and the clergy deals only with the spirit, and the three shall never meet. Because of this incorrect separation, responsible individuals must fill the gaps. The truth is: you are mental, emotional, physical and spiritual beings! What you eat affects your mood, and how you feel about yourself affects your relationship with God. This holy trinity of body, mind and spirit must be integrated into every healing model. No longer can the illusion of separateness be perpetuated. We are all One!

In the field of Mental Health, as in medicine, the healer becomes confined to the area of mental/emotional issues. Nutrition and spirituality were excluded from any of my (Elizabeth), training. I remember when I was working towards my Masters Degree in Mental Health Counseling, I took a marvelous class. The only requirement of this class was that we had to read a preordained number of books, all of which we could choose. Everyone in the class had to discuss the major concepts of three books they had read that week. One evening, I slipped in a very interesting book I read about chakras, which we will discuss later in more detail. During my presentation one of the students made some accusatory remarks about my subject selection, then another student seized the opportunity to chime in. I was amazed that many of my classmates felt it was not okay to discuss chakras in association with counseling. This closed-mindedness serves as a detriment in the medical/mental health field today because it withholds vital information. This is quite unfortunate because, if this information could find its way into the mainstream of Psychology and Psychiatry, many of the patients in mental institutions could be helped as a former patient of mine illustrates.

This middleage man presented himself to me with a variety of complaints ranging from feelings of wanting to tear off his clothes and run naked down the street, to crawling around his house on all fours and barking like a dog. He had numerous phobias and reported talking with the devil. He also kept referring to a fire in his anus that ran up his spine and burned his brain. If you look to the ancient writings of Eastern philosophies it becomes apparent that what this man was describing was the spontaneous rising of the kundalini energy. This energy normally sits dormant in the root chakra or anal area except during orgasm. At that instant of orgasm a very minute part of its potential energy is released resulting in a transient profoundly powerful experience. Who knows how many individuals remain locked away in mental institutions because of an involuntary rise of the kundalini energy which was never explored? The Caudeus, the symbol of snakes intertwining and rising up a staff, symbolizing the practice of medicine, in fact represents the serpent power or kundalini rising up the spinal column. This symbol reminds us that the true role of the healer is not only to relieve the patient from dis- ease but to allow spirit to move through the body with greater ease, transmuting the patient into an enlightened state. This can only occur if the whole patient, as well as the environment surrounding the individual, is examined.

Environmental issues are largely ignored in the treatment of patients. In ancient times the environment was a much simpler issue than today. Religious rituals established a strong bond of love and honor between man, woman and Mother Earth. Today in most modern industrialized nations, individuals are so far removed from nature that this healing bond no longer exists. This lack of respect and disregard for the planet has helped raise environmental issues to new heights resulting in many dis- eases unknown in ancient times.

Environmental factors must also be addressed when facilitating the healing and spiritual evolvement of any patient. If you live in an environment polluted with chemicals, pesticides and 5G electromagnetic waves, your health will be impacted. If you are repressed by your government, financially strapped and under constant stress to survive, spiritual growth will be slowed unless certain basic tools are learned to keep you moving forward. Religioeducative conditioning can also deter personal evolvement by promoting feelings of unworthiness and dependency on others. By identifying each of these areas as potential sources of stagnation in your own spiritual journey, you can decide with greater awareness the path you choose to follow into the future.

When a community, nation, or planet is in a state of '-dis- ease it is the true healers who must first awaken. The call is out for this new breed of healers to first heal themselves. Then they can help facilitate healing within their families, their communities, their countries and the planet.

Physician, Heal Thyself!

Section Two:

The Four Natures

Total wellness is achieved through the environment and integration of all four bodies in your daily life.

CHAPTER 2

PHYSICAL WELLNESS

The moment of conception signals the beginning of the creation of a physical body that will last the incarnating soul a lifetime. This amazing consolidation of billions of cells represents the first of many bodies you possess. The physical body functions at the lowest vibration and is followed in sequence by the emotional, mental and spiritual bodies. To appreciate the true essence of this incredible creation, it helps to see the similarities between the physical body and the cosmos. Now and again a soul dares ask the question, "who am I?" Albert Einstein was one of those souls who theorized electro magnetic forces were responsible for the incredible precision that maintains the Universe in balance. His writings inspired me (Peter), to use my physical body as a reference point and to examine the similarities that exist between myself and the external world. As above, so below, or if you wish, on Earth as it is in Heaven. These powerful phrases symbolize the intricate relationship that exists between you, the microcosm, and the Universe or macrocosm.

Do you ever wonder how it is possible that a human body is capable of such miracles as the conversion of one kind of energy, food for example, into another, muscle? How does it know when and how to heal itself? To be able to see yourself as a composite of billions of cells, trillions of molecules and atoms spinning around each other in perfect harmony just like tiny constellations is mind boggling. The complexity and efficiency of your physical body is indeed amazing. You are a truly three dimensional creation of beauty which houses your equally wondrous spirit. Similarly, one can see the same phenomenon in the Universe where moons spin around planets with stunning precision, planets orbit suns at various speeds, galaxies spin around constellations, and so on into infinity. For every physical law that explains some aspect of how the Universe or macrocosm works, there is a similar law which explains how the same principle works within you, the microcosm.

What is keeping it all together? Why is it that planets do not crash into one another, or into the Sun? When you look into the heavens, you see peace, harmony and beauty. Did you ever wonder why that is so? The answer is love. Love is the cosmic glue that binds the Universe together.

Take a moment to ponder the magnificence of your body. Your physical vehicle is your own private Universe. You have sole ownership of your physical body. The wonderful gift given to you at conception serves as a temple to house your spirit. It is meant to be revered and loved just the way God gave it to you, as a sacred possession, designed to last a lifetime. Understanding this basic truth helps you to appreciate why it is so important to nourish and love your body. Have you ever wondered what keeps your body from falling apart? Love! Do you believe love is a quality that only applies to "living things?" Does a car, a table or a sweater need love? The answer to all these questions is a resounding yes! Love is intelligence, beauty and harmony. Contrary to what most people think love is not an emotion. It is the integrative force that holds every thing in the Universe together.

Both animate and inanimate entities have intelligence. For example, what makes up your body? Tiny particles called atoms that circle around each other. Some of these atoms carry positive charges, some negative charges and still others are neutral. Similarly, a table is made up of many of the same components that you are composed of with some obvious differences. The table seems denser in form and less evolved than you, but does it have an "intelligence?" Yes, it does. For those of you who answered no, take a minute to think. Do you talk to your car? What happens if your car is not maintained or cared for? Will it breakdown and eventually cause you headaches? If you maintain your car by washing it, polishing it, giving it love and attention, your car will last much longer. The same principle applies to any living or inanimate entity including your physical body. Love is the only real truth in this Universe. Therefore, it is understandable that self love is the most important element in healing and evolving your physical body and should be included in everything that enters your body. You are what you drink, eat, breathe and think! It only takes a few moments of contemplation to realize the truth of this statement. Every day when you nourish your body with air, food, water and thoughts, you are demonstrating aspects of self love.

Most everyone knows that the physical body is mostly made up of water molecules. In fact, the planet is mostly water therefore water nutrition is crucial to your physical existence on this planet. Unfortunately, the quality of water has deteriorated over the years. This is especially true in most urban communities where tap water often tastes awful. It is therefore important to purify the water you drink. We only drink purified water and avoid tap water and ice from restaurants and other public places whenever possible. Various water purification systems are available on the market which will provide you with water quality far superior to what most communities can supply.

Other liquid substances like alcohol are detrimental to your body's well being and should be avoided completely. Although alcohol has become a staple in many societies, pharmacologically it acts like any other addicting drug such as cocaine or heroine. It is common knowledge that this powerful drug has irreversible effects on your brain cells as well as your liver metabolism. An even more crucial side effect for those of you interested in spiritual growth, is its potent consequence in lowering the frequency at which you are capable of resonating the cells within your body. We used to include wine with our meals or beer with pizza. Alcoholic drinks were perennially served at every social gathering we attended. Often, after drinking alcohol, we felt tired, depressed and moody. This caused disharmony between us and greatly affected our relationship. We have consequently eliminated all consumption of alcohol or of any other drug from our diet.

As we now observe other individuals who drink regularly, it is easy to spot their lack of clarity and memory lapses. The obvious reason for their noticeable disability is that brain cells are being killed off as they consume this very powerful drug. This goes for drugs of ALL kinds too.

At social gatherings where alcohol is served we are aware that people talk "at" one another, rather than really communicating. Many people depend on alcohol to "break the ice" or need it to "have a good time." Because these people depend on alcohol to foster a false sense of security, they never really develop self confidence. Food nourishment is just as important as water consumption is. Traditionally, you have been taught the significance of eating from the four basic groups of food: carbohydrates, protein, fat and dairy products. Lately, a great deal of information has been disseminated to the public regarding the lethal consequences of consuming foods rich in fats. One of the main dietary sources of fat derives from consuming animal flesh.

Since most people in the United States still eat flesh, I will ask this question: How many of you have visited a slaughter house? I (Peter), did once while growing up. There were several unforgettable characteristics about the place. First, I noticed the cows with their big brown eyes all lined up in single rows waiting inside very narrow corrals to be killed. At the end of this corral was a man holding a gun. His job was to shoot the cows in the head all day long. You could hear the cries miles away as each cow behind the one being killed knew what was about to happen. The smell of the place was also memorable, a unique pungent penetrating odor that persisted in your nostrils. What do you suppose is the predominant thought form in a slaughter house? Fear! Once a thought travels from your mind to your body via the spinal cord, it permeates every cell in your body. This same phenomenon occurs in every living creature. Therefore, the cow about to be killed sends fear, a very powerful disintegrative force, into every cell in its body. Similarly, the fish gasping for oxygen out of the water goes through the same process. The chicken, even if killed as part of a religious ceremony accepted by the Jewish faith (kosher), still experiences the same fear that consequently permeates every cell in its body. When you bite into that steak, chicken, pork loin, fish fillet and so on, you are not only ingesting deadly carcinogens and fat molecules but also fear. You eat the fear which attached itself to every cell of that creature of God as it was being killed. Fear affects your thought patterns, behavior and general health. It's no wonder fear is the predominate thought form on this planet.

What about vegetables? Do they have an intelligence also? Yes, they do. Is the plant kingdom as evolved as the animal kingdom? No, it is not. A major difference between the ingestion of a vegetable and of an animal is that most often the plant is not killed when eaten but continues to grow. However, in the case of roots, saying a short prayer prior to ingesting it is sufficient to erase any negative karma (Universal Law of Cause and Effect).

Each soul has the right to express itself. When you shorten the life of an animal by eating its flesh, it loses the right of self expression. This act becomes a karmic debt incurred by you that must be repaid. Karmically what goes around comes around, therefore flesh eaters are known to have more heart attacks, strokes, breast and intestinal cancers and other chronic debilitating medical conditions than vegetarians. In our home we made the decision several years ago to become vegetarians. As a physician, I (Peter), recognized several biological facts that give the proper clues as to our vegetarian origin. Compared to carnivorous creatures our intestinal tract is physically too long. Our hands are made to gather foods rather than to tear flesh. We sweat to keep cool instead of panting like carnivorous animals do, and so on.

Logistically, for us as vegetarians living in a flesh, oriented society, the main difficulty has been in finding a nutritious selection of foods to eat when we travel. Many restaurants use meat products in preparing vegetables and legumes, so it is in your best interest to ask how your food is prepared before putting it into your body. Hopefully, one day restaurants will be forced to list all ingredients on their menus. When grocery shopping we have learned to carefully read labels not only for fat content but also for animal products such as egg whites and gelatin often found in so called "vegetarian" products but also for sugar products, artificial chemicals, and GMO (genetically modified organisms and for animal products such as egg whites and gelatin often found in so called "vegetarian" products. We found it is best to buy fresh fruits and vegetables from your local farmers, or better yet grow your own and set up a community co-op for trading! Make everything from scratch it tastes better and you know what you are putting in your mouth. A high vibrational diet including lot's of live fresh fruits and vegetables brings you LIFE! Eggs are not only unhealthy to consume because of the high cholesterol content, but also symbolize life itself and should be eliminated from your diet. Realizing the typical American diet is centered around flesh and eggs, it is important to give some general guidelines as to what is a healthy diet. With few exceptions, the perfect diet is one rich in carbohydrates and low in protein and fat. Dairy products, beans, lentils, spinach and kale, just to name a few, are excellent sources of protein. Certain individuals do well eating dairy products while others do not. Milk and all its derivatives are classified as rich foods and can be highly allergenic. The fat content in most of these products is also unacceptably high for anyone concerned about his/her weight. The ingestion of beans and lentils can cause flatulence in some individuals while others thrive on them. As you learn to develop your intuitive awareness it will become easier to identify your body type and what your needs are at various stages of your evolvement.

I (Elizabeth), have learned that we are all electrochemical beings with unique and diverse compositions. This explains the old saying "one person's medicine is another person's poison." The most important things is to learn to listen to your body to determine its moment to moment needs. You don't have to remain locked into one specific diet that becomes like a religion to you, but can make adjustments according to your bodies current needs. By determining your unique body needs, you can then create a full menu around it. An ancient but still valid medical science which describes the different body types is Ayuverdic medicine. Our bibliography includes several books where you may read more about this fascinating field of nutritional medicine.

At present the greatest threat to our health is the ever increasing levels of toxicity on our planet. This is generated by a combination things which work together including the metals and nanotechnology found in the food we eat, water we drink and air we breath; the chemtrails, which work with the toxic radiation levels emitted 5G weaponry and the destructive electro magnetism generated from the Space X Satellite Cage now surrounding our planet. This combined with the bio technology now inside many human hosts creates a very toxic cocktail. Protecting yourself from the high levels of toxic radiation is a key factor in maintaining your health. This may include relocating to avoid toxic environments, heavy populated areas and using technology responsibly by unplugging and shielding your devices and protecting your home and family. It is imperative to create a healing home environment and sleep sanctuary and use wisdom when you must interact with toxic people, places or things. You must also maintain a healthy inner environment inside your physical body by detoxing the metals from your body daily and maintaining a high PH Balance of 7.35 to 7.45 level. Alkalizing your body is key. Baking Soda is an effective way to immediately Alkalize your body but it should be followed by an Alkaline Diet using an abundance of live fruits and vegetables.

Most commercial farming relies on the use of herbicides, fungicides and pesticides to grow their crops. These toxic substances do not wash off with plain water but are incorporated into the molecular structure of ordinary produce. Now we have the GMO (genetically modified organisms) taking over of our world's industrial farming. These genetically modified fruits and vegetables do not give your body the nutrients it needs and genetically modifies your body. Insects won't touch these food. Because of the potential health hazard in consuming these contaminated foods, it is in your best interest to purchase locally grown organic produce whenever possible. Through Food Coops many communities are now offering an ever increasing variety of privately grown organic produce and meat analogues (totally vegetarian foods that have the consistency of meat such as the veggie burger). These products make a vegetarian diet incredibly delicious and nutritious as well as allowing you to evolve some old fashion recipes you were raised on. However it is becoming very important to know what exactly they are putting in these fake meat products. Many are filled with artificial and genetically modified ingredients hazardous to your health. If these facilities are not available in your area, you should ask your grocer to include organic produce in their store. Your grocer may be reluctant to add organic products to his/her store and cite several excuses such as: "commercially grown fruits and vegetables taste the same to most people, or they are too expensive for most customers." The issue here is not taste but quality. Do you want toxins in your body? Though it is true that these products are more expensive, they are well worth the extra cost.

Caffeine is another substance that interferes with our concentration and meditations. Sometime ago I (Peter), also became aware of how it effected my heart rhythm and surgical skills. Thus, I have also omitted most caffeine—containing products from my daily regimen. Consumption of sugar and chocolate is a sensitive area. Many individuals have been taught that these substances are harmful. Like anything else, too much of one thing can carry health consequences. Sugar is a product that which can cause many health issues . For those who enjoy deserts (and who doesn't) natural organic sugar substitutes can make life more enjoyable. We enjoy fresh organic stevia leaves. It brings a certain quality of sweetness to life and chocolate warms the heart! By substituting healthy alternatives , I (Elizabeth), have been able to reproduce almost any dessert.

Moderation is the key to ingesting these controversial food products. Dietary supplementation is another area that deserves some attention. Our opinion is that most of us are not receiving the full complement of vitamins and minerals in the foods we eat. Several years ago we began to take a vegetarian vitamins and minerals , herbs, and several grams of vitamin C a day and other antioxidants a daily DETOX and periodic herbal and parasite cleansing. Detoxifying your body daily is the name of the game and in many cases necessary to maintain your physical body in our world today. Find what works for you. We drink herbal cleansing teas both hot and cold. I (Elizabeth) us Wormwood daily it is an excellent cure for most everything especially parasites. Working up good sweat is great for detoxing your body. Saunas, stream rooms, hot springs, or just siting in the Sun can do wonders. Lymphatic drainage, Exfoliating your skin and invigorating your circulation are key components. I suggest you do your own research and find out which daily practices your body likes best and fit into your lifestyle. This routine has proven to be immensely helpful to us in evolving our physical vehicles especially since our environment continues to deteriorate. As important as what you drink and eat is what you breathe.Air is essential to life. The quality of our air has become a global issue. Clean fresh air is difficult to come by these days.

Every breath you take sustains you for a few seconds before you must fill your lungs again with a new breath. The quality of the air you breathe varies a great deal from place to place. Most indoor workplaces today are air conditioned. To condition air you mostly remove the humidity and cool it. True conditioning would be to pass the air through a series of filters to remove pollutants or even viral particles that can affect your health. Few places today pay attention to the quality of the air their employees breathe eight to ten hours a day. The harmful effects of passive smoking are becoming quite clear to health providers. It matters little if your place of employment allows smoking in certain areas but not others. Unless a separate air-conditioning system is provided to the smoking areas, eventually everyone breathes the same carcinogens. If you are one of the many individuals who work indoors, I suggest passing around a petition to alert other coworkers of the potential health hazards of breathing polluted air and requesting that management upgrade the air quality of your office. This is also true of other public places such as restaurants where smokers and nonsmokers are all placed in one huge room. Now we have a new enemy to our health and that is the mandated which has become a habitual wearing of surgical masks. Many people think of it as a permanent part of their anatomy. (Elizabeth) I have seen new borns fitted with masks shortly after taking their first breath of life. How can you properly throw out toxins, and breath in clean life giving air wearing a mask? How can you relax and access higher states of consciousness conducive to healing?

While on the topic of breathing a few words about the importance of proper breathing techniques should be said. Five minutes of forced inhalation/exhalation exercises a day is equivalent to running a mile. Diaphragmatic breathing will release toxins and immediately revitalize every cell in your body with oxygen and prana (the life force that permeates the Universe). In other words, there is a lot more to breathing than simply taking a breath.

Included in the categories of unseen air pollutants we need to say a few words about manmade electromagnetic waves, especially 5G and up. These invisible waves of energy have also been identified as a tremendous source of health hazards, in particular to those individuals who live in congested areas and near power lines. Scientists and epidemiological data demonstrates a link between C.O.V.I.D. (Certification OF Vaccination Identification Documentation) certain rare as well as cancers and a host of other dis-eases are linked to electromagnetic waves especially 5G. Intuition will tell you that the human race is not meant to live in overpopulated areas where your body is constantly being bombarded from every direction by air pollutants, water contaminants and food supplies poisoned by the extensive use of fungicides, herbicides, pesticides, hormones and other chemicals.

Equally important to eating, drinking, and breathing is physical fitness. Physical fitness is an integral part of maintaining a healthy body. It is important to exercise and stretch regularly to keep your muscles and joints in perfect working condition and increase your breathing capacity by performing cardiovascular exercises that allow the body to take in more air or Prana. It is vital to exercise daily, whether this activity comes from walking, running, hiking, biking, dancing, swimming or whatever your favorite activity may be. The object is to speed up your heart rate to exercise its muscle layers and increase the blood supply to itself. As difficult as it may be to accomplish this goal for those of you who keep a busy schedule, it is of the utmost importance. I (Elizabeth), recommend walking. In many cultures walking is in an integral part of daily life. Instead of taking one long walk—spread your walking out. Walk in the morning, after each meal and in the evening, even if it is only for twelve minutes at a time. Walk to work or around the neighborhood. In changing seasons, dress warmly and enjoy the elements of wind, rain and snow. If it is too much for you, buy a walker and do it indoors, or go to a mall. Once you incorporate a simple exercise routine into your daily schedule it should not be hard to make exercise a part of your day. Many places of employment are now offering such health oriented programs. Hopefully, health insurance carriers will give reduced premium rates to those who promote physical fitness.

Even if you follow the perfect vegetarian diet I described earlier, eventually you may be faced with another problem obesity. Obesity has become quite common in the past twenty-five years. There are at least several factors that can be identified playing a role in this phenomenon. Becoming a sedentary individual or "couch potato" adds to the problem. Obesity is the result of trying to feed all four natures at the physical level only. You must realize the importance of nurturing all four of your natures. This is the primary reason why most ordinary diets do not work: they only address the single issue of losing physical weight. Overweight individuals need to face a greater reality if they are to succeed in permanently keeping lean and healthy. A lasting change will begin to take place when they learn that it is only through the proper maintenance of your physical vehicle and its loving care and treatment that your body will last a lifetime.

Have you ever wondered why home cooking tastes so good? The reason is that it has a very special ingredient: love. You mentally energize the food with loving thoughts while preparing the meal. Do you eat out frequently? What energy is common to many restaurants? People are busy. Do you believe the people who work there are taking the time to add that special ingredient called love? If they are, I guarantee you the food will taste better. The preparation of a meal should be done as a moving meditation. As much as possible, take your time to prepare the meal and be consciously aware of the energy you are putting into what you are preparing. Be in the present moment. If you have guests, get them involved during the preparation of the meal or setting the table. As they join in, you will immediately feel a shift in the energies and I guarantee everyone will enjoy the food tremendously. When you sit at the table, you may want to play soft music in the background to put you in the mood to receive. The next step is to quiet yourself and pay respects to Mother Earth and all those souls who contributed to the meal, starting with the farmer who planted and harvested the crop, the driver who brought it to the store and all who prepared the meal. You could thank the plant kingdom for providing the vegetables and the animal kingdom for giving you the dairy products you enjoy eating. Focus on the food as you eat it, feel it nourishing your body.

After eating, the washing of the dishes can be just as spiritual as the meal itself. Remember, everything you do is spiritual, even moving your bowels which happens to be a cleansing process to remove impurities from your body. It is only when you blind yourself with limiting beliefs and judgements that you keep from seeing the spirituality of all things. Just as you must bring your spirituality into your physical body, so must you integrate your emotional and mental bodies. Emotional and mental nourishment through correct thinking is as important in maintaining physical wellness as water, food and air.

Your thoughts create emotional feelings that form physical responses within your body. Think of a time when someone you loved said they were leaving you. Did you feel the energy drain down your body and into your feet? Just as thoughts affect your physical wellness, so can manifestations of 'dis- ease in your body be clues as to what may be going on in your life at the emotional/ mental level.

If you are suffering from an ailment, ask yourself a few questions until you get an "Aha" as to why a particular illness has manifested. Here are some examples:

Headaches: Are you thinking too much?

Sinus: Could this be pressure to see something in your life?

Throat: (which happens to be the seat of the will) Have you said something you regret? Are you giving up your will or not accepting nurturing?

Lung Congestion: Where in your life are you suffocating?

Heart: Do you have a broken heart?

Liver: Are you the town dump? Does everyone bring their problems to you? Are you angry?

Constipation: Are you holding on to old business, old hurts and blames?

Hemorrhoids: Is something following you around? Overweight: Are you carrying around excess baggage? Knees: Do you need others to support you?

Overweight: Are you carrying around excess baggage?

Knees: Do you need others to support you?

Feet: Do you lack a solid foundation?

'Dis- ease serves as a signal that something needs attending to in other areas of your life. As you learn to properly care for your physical vehicle, you will release stress from every cell in your body and bring your emotions into balance.

CHAPTER 3
EMOTIONAL WELLNESS

The next level up from the physical body in vibrational frequency is the emotional body, which in the human form is intimately related to the physical body. Humans have often been described as emotional creatures. Frequently emotions become an addiction because the individual's will is taken over by the animal part of the soul. This aspect of the soul works from an instinctual level responding to external stimuli in much the same way as a wild creature. By comparison, the Godsoul aspect is linked to the higher self and the Universal mind, giving you limitless potential.

This links you to more evolved human attributes such as love and compassion for self and others and true knowledge.

"It's just emotion that's taking me over," are the profound lyrics to a popular tune by the Bee gees, best describing how emotions often become the roller coaster ride of life. During a typical day, how often do you find yourself giving way to your emotions? Are you in control of your emotions or are they in control of you?

Because of the close relationship that exists between the physical and emotional bodies, havoc is in store for those who cannot control their emotions. In dis- eases such as ulcers, migraine headaches, irritable bowel syndrome, insomnia and asthma, it is easy to see how emotional dis- ease translates into physical dis- ease. The truth is, if ignored, all emotional dis-eases will eventually manifest in the physical body. Ease the emotional turmoil and you will ease the body.

A patient I treated a few years ago illustrates this strong mind-body-dis-ease connection. Sarah was a twenty-seven year old female who came to the office complaining of weight loss. According to the patient, the weight loss began nine months earlier following the unexpected death of her baby two weeks prior to the due date. Up to that point the pregnancy had progressed quite normally until one day she did not feel the baby move.

Apparently the dead baby had been delivered by cesarean leaving her with not only a physical scar, but a deep emotional scar as well. Several psychotherapists had prescribed drugs to help relieve her constant state of despair. The patient wept frequently, expressing anger at God for having taken her baby while suffering from a tremendous feeling of guilt. She was convinced that somehow God had punished her for having done something wrong. To make matters worse, her current relationship was on the verge of collapse because of her constant state of depression.

Though she hoped to heal some of her grief with another pregnancy, she dared not go through with it because a therapist had advised against it. Totally out of control, she felt life was closing in on her and she was ready to give it up.

As difficult as it must be to accept events such as the one effecting my former patient, one way to make the acceptance easier is to realize all life experiences are placed along your path for self discovery and spiritual unfoldment. Only those with expanded awareness can understand the highest meaning of why things happen.

Until you have such awareness you can only speculate and trust that the experience was not an accident and the soul who chose that particular infant's body knew ahead of time the outcome of the pregnancy. By helping the patient gain a greater sense of awareness into the complete meaning of this event, she could begin the healing process.

Uncontrolled emotions can harm people and destroy property as graphically illustrated in today's media. Every day, newspapers are filled with stories of how individuals permanently changed their lives in a single moment of despair, jealousy or rage. We have seen angry girlfriends burn boyfriends' estates, husbands kill their wives, mothers murder their own children and so on. It appears that many individuals have reached an emotional boiling point, frequently victimizing their loved ones.

Our nation's social unrest, fueled by emotions and turmoil, can be as destructive as a major natural disaster. Riots leave extensive property damage and loss of life. They are a graphic illustration of how racial tension, combined with years of oppression, can explode like puss bursting out of an infected wound so that the healing process may take place. Often an emotional outpouring is the first step toward healing, much the same way the body throws off toxins while repairing itself. Emotional pain can also motivate the individual to change destructive behavioral patterns. But if left unchecked these patterns will keep you stuck in the never ending roller coaster ride of anger, rage, jealousy, hate, self pity, shame, etc. As an evolving soul on a spiritual path, your job is to rise above the animal part of your soul that causes you to react emotionally to external stimuli rather than remaining peacefully centered and internally focused. Emotions such as fear, lust and anger lower your vibrational frequency and feed the illusion of separateness from God. But you must first feel your emotions to heal your emotions. We all hold trauma, pain and sorrow within our body tissue. By allowing yourself to feel this trauma you can you detox them out your body's cellar memory. Then and only then can you transmute these base emotions.

According to the law of Karma, for every action there must be an equal or opposite reaction. Take the example of a heroin addict who will experience a low of equal proportion to the high he felt after his last fix. As the addiction becomes stronger it eventually occupies his/her life. As the will is consumed by the drug, his/her physical body begins to pay back the karmic debt s/he accrued by living an unnatural and unbalanced existence. Instead of functioning from a peaceful center, the individual finds her/himself a victim to his/her own actions swinging from one emotional extreme to the next. The same principle applies to everyday situations if you allow yourself to be controlled by the external world. The external world, like a drug, can give an individual emotional highs and lows to the point where s/he is constantly looking outside him/herself for emotional fulfillment much the same way the addict looks towards a drug. At first glance, it may be difficult to appreciate this analogy, but if examined carefully one can readily see the similarities.

Let us look at Frank, a used car salesperson who on a particular day felt the joy of everything going right for him. He made a few sales that earned him the admiration of his friends and coworkers. This was a great day. Dependent upon the external world to supply him with his sense of self esteem, Frank felt good because of external conditions. This is Frank's high. The next day, Frank realized nobody wanted to buy his cars. His coworkers ignored him. Because of his dependency on the external world for his sense of well being, Frank felt depressed as his emotions dragged him down. This was Frank's low.

Although not as extreme, it is easy to recognize that the highs and lows of a heroine addict and an emotional addict are alike in many respects. By placing your focus outside yourself you leave the door wide open for the ups and downs of life. The pathway off the emotional roller coaster is to be in it, but not of it. This means be in the world going about your business, but not in it to the extent that you become hooked on the emotional ride. This is the key to emotional wellness. The way to accomplish this task is to bring the focus inward. As you do this, life can be viewed with a greater sense of objectivity much like watching a movie. As you can look at life from an inward focus, you will become more detached and less affected by the outcome of life's events. In this way you can move beyond the pull of emotions.

This is not to be confused with burying or hiding emotions. Painful issues need to be brought into the light, like puss that oozes from a sore, to help you move through the experience. One problem men often face is the shutting off of their emotions, since it has been deemed socially unacceptable for them to be emotional. The reason becoming detached and removing yourself from the emotional roller coaster of life becomes so tricky is that you must first feel to become whole to evolve past the pull of emotions. To become whole you must satisfy all your unfulfilled desires. This can be done in a simple fashion. You may desire to become a pilot but could feel satisfaction by simply taking a single flying lesson. You may long to live in a palace but taking a tour of one is enough to satisfy your soul's desire. Remember, the point is to fulfill the desires so that you may free yourself from them. Desires are the chains that bind you to Maya, the world of illusions.

Through the magic of movies, modern technology can transport us to any time or space. Why do you think movies are so popular in today's culture? In ancient Greece it was believed that an audience experienced an emotional catharsis as they participated in the telling of a story by way of the theatrical event. The audience grew from the experience and released their emotions as if they had experienced it themselves. Movies allow the audience to see the devastating effects revenge, jealousy, guilt and rage have upon a person's life, without having to personally live through those experiences. In this manner movies can be seen as another vehicle to help you satisfy your desires.

There is a tendency for individuals to linger in an emotional experience rather than to let it go and move on to the next thing. Chances are these people re-live the same experience over and over again. By placing your focus on the past, you will miss opportunities that present themselves to you. The past is gone and the future is now, so allow yourself the freedom and spontaneity of operating in the present moment. Learn to live in the present!

As you review your life, what events, people, or things are you still attached to? In what areas of your life do you feel there is something you cannot do without? Is it a relationship, money, social status, alcohol, tobacco, food or sex? Unfortunately, in a misguided attempt to reach inner peace, many souls have turned to pharmaceutical companies to numb their minds with tranquilizers, sleeping pills and other over the counter products. Any product or service that is in some way related to stress reduction is in great demand. Though people long for peacefulness, they are looking in the wrong places. Peace begins (and ends) within yourself.

In the Eastern culture equanimity (evenness of mind) becomes necessary in reaching Nirvana (oneness with God). At this level of awareness the spiritual seeker can remove personal judgement from ordinary life events thus remaining in a true state of peacefulness.

An ancient metaphor told to us by a friend which illustrates this philosophy is the story of a Chinese farmer who lived in a small village where his daily ritual was to meet his friends at the tea house at sunset. The farmer owned a mare that ran off one day leaving him without a horse to work the fields. That evening he shared the news with his friends who reacted by saying "Your mare ran off? Oh, that is very bad. How will you work the field?" The next day the farmer's mare came home bringing a beautiful stallion with her. That afternoon the farmer went back to the tea house and shared the news. "She brought a stallion back? Oh that is very good, now you can have more horses to work the farm."

The next day the farmer's only son broke his leg while breaking in the stallion. That afternoon the farmer went back to the tea house and told his friends. "Oh that is bad. Since you have no other sons, you'll have to do all the work yourself." A few days later a man from the military came to the village and took away all the young men to fight in the war, all except the farmer's son, whose leg was broken. That afternoon the farmer went back to the tea house and his friends said "Your son was not taken to the war? Oh that is good, soon he'll be able to harvest your field and all your neighbors' fields which will make you a rich man."

This simple story shows how people are constantly judging life events as either good or bad, when the fact is, things just happen! From most individuals limited perspective, it is impossible to know the true meaning of an event except to realize that there are no accidents. Instead of letting your ego analyze, categorize and judge these experiences, why not allow yourself to explore the highest meaning of life's events and learn in the process how to surrender yourself to God.

As discussed in the chapter on physical wellness, an intimate relationship between body and mind is maintained through electrochemical neurotransmitters that quickly convert a sensory input into an appropriate bodily response (or inappropriate depending on how well the individual can control his emotions). Living in a constant state of emotional turmoil exemplified by fear, anger and despair, will destroy the delicate balance that maintains wellness in your physical body. As you continue to abuse the body dis- eases such as insomnia, ulcers, heart dis- ease and even cancer can take their toll.

Fear is the predominant thought form on our planet. Fear is a very powerful and immobilizing force. Often fear clouds the perception of events that present themselves along an individual's path. In any disaster it is generally the ones who panic that end up losing their lives or making the crisis worse. Ironically, fear does not help. Instead it acts as a magnifying lens, making things worse than they really are. Ask anyone and they will say the most important thing to do in any crisis is to remain calm and not lose your head. Take a moment out of your day and observe how many decisions you make based on fear. In relationships, are you being motivated by fear of abandonment? Are you fearful about losing your job, or do you think your children will stop loving you if you discipline them? Are you afraid God will punish you if you do not go to church on Sundays? Frequently individuals are willing to give up huge amounts of personal freedom for the illusion that something or someone bigger and stronger than they are will protect them. This someone may be a spouse, a parent, a religion or even a government. The truth is, it is only by rising above your fears and using your intuitive powers that you can take care of your self. Intuition, unpolluted by fear, is the best means of caring for yourself.

Stories abound regarding individuals who sensed impending disaster and refused to get in a car, on a plane, or called someone to warn them about something they believed was going to happen. Intuition is the only real way of taking care of yourself in these turbulent times. Fear is like a loud overpowering tape recording blasting out in your head, while your intuition is a very subtle and sweet melody much like a symphony of violins. In order to listen, you must first quite down the loud and unrelenting "fear tape" to best tune into the subtleties of your intuitive voice. When individuals first learn to listen to their in-tuition they may mistake their fears for intuitive messages and misjudge events and lose faith in themselves. You must keep practicing just as you do when flexing a new set of muscles. Ceasing the consumption of fear in the form of flesh will help.

Have you ever been in a very peaceful space only to find that the minute you are around other people you tend to pick up their emotional state? Thoughts are things. They are powerful unseen forces that you can easily tap into depending on your state of mind. Everything in the Universe can be expressed in terms of energy.

Imagine yourself as a receiver and transmitter of energy waves. In the case of love, powerful integrative energy waves emanate from your aura, permeating those around you. Conversely, fear waves will similarly reach your aura and either bounce back and ground themselves elsewhere or permeate the space between your cells, thus affecting your behavior. This phenomenon explains why you feel peaceful in certain places and ill at ease in others. After a while these thought forms assume a life of their own and affect those who come in contact with them. As you learn to maintain equanimity and surround yourself with love, the emotions emanating from these thought forms will not affect you. By remaining in a one point focus and retaining your own precious energy, you will soon develop the ability to glide through most human experiences that used to throw you into chaos.

It is important to learn how to recognize the energy in certain places and how to conduct yourself in these areas so that you are not drawn into them. Keep your own precious energy and avoid leaving yourself wide open for these unforeseen forces.

In the Western hemisphere individuals tend to talk too much, frequently revealing personal matters to anyone who is willing to listen. Next time this happens try letting the person next to you tell their story. Instead of talking, just listen. This will give you a better opportunity to observe yourself and your emotions. The individual will leave thinking you're the nicest person in the world. Likewise, on a non physical level, pay attention to the energy in the places you visit and sense what thought forms are there. Focus on the reason you are there. If you are conducting business, get the job done and leave as quickly as possible. Do not linger.

As you evolve into operating from a place of equanimity, from time to time something may push your "button" and momentarily throw you back into the grips of emotional turmoil. Not to worry. This does not negate all the progress you have made thus far. Nor does it give you license to start beating yourself up emotionally. This is simply a little test. The minute you realize your mistake, change it! Get off the roller coaster as quickly as possible. One way to do this is to focus on your breathing pattern. Then say the words, "I am" as you inhale, feeling the air flow into your nose, down your windpipe. As you exhale through your mouth say the words "peace," letting the air warm your heart. Keep repeating, "I am...peace. I am... peace." After a few moments you will notice your body relaxing and soon your breathing will become slower and deeper. Before long you will be at peace again. Or perhaps you just want to lighten up and laugh at yourself or find something amusing about the situation. Take a moment to get out of your head. The intellect can be a relentless entrapment. Take a moment to still you brain. Walk in nature. Turn off the internal chatter.

When you have regained your state of equanimity take a moment to look deeper into the event that triggered you. What was it that aggravated the little child within you? Was it a deep underlying feeling of fear? Abandonment? Shame? Guilt? Unworthiness? Powerlessness? Keep digging until you can get to the root cause of it. Then look at where in your life did this event first happen? Who was there? Are you still buying into these sinful (incorrect beliefs) about yourself and the world around you? Then take some kind of action to change your thoughts, then your emotions and you will heal and your triggers will melt away. The human journey back toward its original state of Godliness is like a hike up a mountain. It may become treacherous in spots and requires moments of rest. Don't be afraid to take a rest period and start again when your energy returns. Remember, all pathways lead Home (Oneness with God).

Often when people encounter obstacles or deterrents in everyday life their reaction is to roll up their sleeves and force an issue. I think back on an old song "If it don't fit, don't force it. Just relax and let it flow. Just cause that's how you want it doesn't mean it should be so." When this happens realize it is your ego that is trying to control you. Take a step away and refocus by gathering your energy and try another approach, only softer this time. If the problem persists, let it go. It is not for you to do or solve. Often it becomes an issue of timing and nothing more. As you learn to surrender yourself to God, you quickly realize nothing happens until it is supposed to happen.

Similarly, by learning to say no and to not be "nice" saves you much wasted time and pain. Before participating in an activity ask yourself this question, "Is this furthering my progress along my spiritual path?" If the answer is no, don't do it. This does not mean you should go around being nasty to people. But it allows you to simply become more focused. It's a lot easier to say no than to deal with the consequences of a wrong action. Remember the law of Karma.

In the case of "saving" someone, remember the old saying "rescuers become victims." The next time you jump in to help someone, be careful. If that moment is for you, then do your job and get out clean. For example, if a small child falls and breaks his leg and you're the only person on the street, that experience is meant for you. Help the child, comfort him/her until the paramedics arrive, then go on your way. You've done your job. Don't go out looking to save people, but if a fellow human being extends a needy hand, help them and move on. The problem with trying to save victims who say they want help is that no matter what you do or say they often will reject or negate what you offer. Although you may hold the answer for them, they are not in the time or space to receive it. Somewhere along the line you can hope that they will be ready and that another soul will come along and give them the input they need. It is not your responsibility.

As you grow new eyes and ears coming from a high place of spiritual awareness, your service to self and others can begin. You will meet the needs of soul rather than the wants of ego by coming from a place of true compassion. Pitying or joining others in their sorrow will not help. Instead, be a guiding light capable of generating a loving and healing presence by releasing your emotions and operating from your mental body.

CHAPTER 4
MENTAL WELLNESS

The next step up in the vibrational scale from the emotional body is the mental body. In its purest form the mental body functions as pure thought directly connected to spirit which is unhindered by emotion. When this occurs only joy and bliss permeate the physical body. By learning to integrate your physical, emotional and mental bodies you then become self-realized. You are here on the "earth campus" to achieve this exalted state of being. As you arrive on the campus there are certain courses being offered. Depending on your own life agenda, you must learn in much the same way a university student chooses a curriculum. There are five basic courses. Most individuals are running all five of them at the same time.

The five basic courses are: not knowing your own personal power, feelings of unworthiness, being too sensitive, or not being sensitive enough, and overcoming fear.

Thoughts direct energy. If improperly directed they are capable of manifesting dis- ease in the physical body. Not long ago I (Peter), treated a patient with multiple physical and emotional complaints illustrating the concept of thoughts improperly directing energy. My patient was fortysix years old and divorced from an alcoholic husband who abused her in many different ways. After the examination I told her many of her physical problems (obesity, depression, insomnia, hyper tension, headaches, etc.) were due to negligence of her physical body. She responded "Doctor, I was taught that you live for your husband and children. Well, I don't have a husband anymore and my two daughters are grown and don't care about me. The truth is, I don't have a life."

This patient typifies the significance of thoughts directing energy in a self destructive manner. Totally lacking self esteem, the patient lived a life of selfinduced punishment. She had reached the point where nothing was left except a very unhappy soul trapped within a decaying middleaged body. Meanwhile, she continued to torment herself because of belief systems she learned as a child that negated her self worth and ultimately manifested in multiple physical illnesses.

To evolve mentally you must be willing to examine every belief system you have developed and every thought pattern that you have adopted. Then you must have the courage to discard any belief that stands in the way of your complete evolvement. Through this cleansing process a new sense of awareness will emerge. Often beliefs are so well hidden within the personality self that they escape the individual's consciousness unless a recurring behavioral pattern that leads to disharmony is closely scrutinized. These belief systems are "borrowed" from parents, educators, religious teachers and society at large. After a while these beliefs become your own often leading to disharmony, unhappiness and dis- ease. Many people define themselves according to their beliefs. For example, I'm a Catholic, a Republican, a lawyer and so on. You become so entrenched in your belief system you begin to miss the forest for the trees. The truth is you are God.

I (Elizabeth), remember reading a case study in graduate school concerning a patient who had a multiple personality disorder. One of her personalities was deathly allergic to oranges. If she ate even a small bite of an orange she would break out in hives. However, another one of her personalities loved oranges and demonstrated no physical ill effects from their consumption. The mind can kill you or heal you, depending on how your thoughts are directed. It can bring you closer to God and your true self or it can lead you into darkness, despair and suffering. The choice is yours.

How is it that individuals accumulate beliefs and spend most of their lives operating from them, never once questioning their usefulness? I am reminded of a story about a young woman who always cut the top part off a ham before putting it into a baking pan. One day curiosity struck and she asked her mother why she always cut the top off the ham. Her mother laughed and told her it was because her pan was too small so she had to cut it in half so that it would fit.

A great number of individuals are so angry with their parents for all the terrible things they did when raising them. The truth is, you chose your parents before incarnating for old business, new business, body type and various other courses you needed to complete. Those souls were simply following the "butt" in front of them; that is, adopting beliefs from their own parents. For generations humans, have followed the sets of beliefs handed down to them by their parents, never questioning if there was indeed a better way of doing things. Look at your life. Do you eat what your parents eat? Live where your parents live? Practice the same religion your parents practice? Raise your children the same way you were raised? To what extent are you still following the "butt" in front of you? If you are to evolve, you must be willing to recreate yourself anew. You must think in new categories and have the courage to live life according to your own rules as you follow your unique purpose. Perhaps there are certain family beliefs that can be summarized by sayings about your family, "We Mulligans are a tough bunch," or favorite stories that dead ancestors have passed on which accumulate energy through the years. Perhaps you hold on to beliefs associated with your social class, skin color, religion, sexual preference, nationality or gender. The extent to which you are attached to your beliefs is the extent to which you hold yourself back. In other words, you are one belief away from being Godrealized.

Your emotions are intricately connected to your perceptions of things. Let's look at the story of the Chinese farmer told in the chapter on emotional wellness. When the day's events were judged as bad the emotional response was negative; when judged as good, the response was positive. Change your perception of the event and you change the emotional response. Once you have managed to free yourself from disharmonious thoughts and patterns then you can rise above the limitations of your brain and begin to experience true bliss and wisdom. Wisdom does not come from intellectual bantering but from the stillness of knowing.

In the West we tend to spend too much time in our heads. To achieve mental wellness you need to park your degrees outside the door and become as little children, knowing with your heart, instead of reasoning with your mind. Get out of your head! You must cease the relentless chatter of your brain and allow yourself to be nurtured by stillness. In the creation of the Universe everything evolved from stillness. This is your way of paying homage to the Creator and reminding yourself of your spiritual origin. As you learn to become still new levels of awareness and knowledge will be reached with patience and the passage of linear time.

Mental wellness is one of the four natures you must develop in your human condition. Modern life is full of distractions, so it is not uncommon to frequently find yourself in the midst of a storm of stimuli constantly testing your will to remain calm and peacefully centered.

Self criticism is another activity many of you find yourselves engaged in. Critical messages from your parents stay with you long after you leave home. These limiting beliefs can keep you from loving yourself and moving freely in the world with confidence and awareness. Similarly, beliefs about sin, unworthiness and guilt undermine and sabotage your soul's complete unfoldment. You must learn to fully accept the truth that you are loved and are part of God, beautiful and unique in your own way. You are here to learn and grow, not to suffer and be punished. Each and every one of you is worthy to receive an abundance of good things! By criticizing yourself and others, by always seeing the glass half empty, rather than half full, you are cheating yourself of your birthright to experience joy, love and gratitude. When you see the best in others, you bring out the best in yourself. When you create negative energy patterns, they travel out into the Universe and boomerang back to you. However, if you radiate love and gratitude it will come back to you tenfold. When you catch yourself in a pattern of negativity, stop where you are and change the energy immediately. You'll find your whole day, and perhaps your life, will change. To evolve along your spiritual path you must be willing to let go of old hurts and blames.

Often anger, despair and other negative thoughts come from misperceptions as the ego filters in only pieces of information depending on your belief systems. Take the example of a couple riding in a train. Each one is looking out a window on opposing sides of the train. On one side there are forests, mountains and streams. On the other side are deserts, rocks, and canyons. One person's reality is different from the other. You will have different perceptions of things. Just accept that as a fact and do not waste your time trying to convince another of your opinion.

Mental wellness also involves taking responsibility for yourself and letting go of the responsibility for others. Often people feel responsible for all sorts of things outside themselves. If their child is not doing well in school, it's their fault. If their spouse is angry, it's their fault. Our society tends to want to make other people responsible. Similarly, many individuals tend to blame others for their own shortcomings. Like little children they wait for mother or father to come and make it better, rather than taking control of their lives and empowering themselves to change. You have the power to change your entire life. It is simply a moment to moment choice.

I (Peter), recall a day I spent at our cottage on Captiva Island in Florida. As usual I awoke early in the morning and drank two cups of coffee (decaffeinated) made from some new beans I was trying out and grabbed my beach chair, towel, sunglasses, suntan lotion and briefcase and headed to the beach. The shoreline was just a short walk from the little cottage. The sight of the sea was unusually breathtaking: Still emerald waves lapped at the shore dissolving into an indigo blue that shimmered off into the horizon. Seagulls, pelicans, great blue herons and ospreys were eating their breakfast around me. Two pigeons dancing in the art of their lovemaking, were startled by my movement. Litter from an overturned garbage pail signaled that my raccoon friends had feasted on left over pasta and beans. What a beautiful day this was! What a miracle that I had turned my life around enough to recognize its beauty! A true sense of mental wellness filled every cell of my body. By changing my perception of the world I had allowed myself this joyous moment. "Was it that simple?" I thought. It was. My perception of the world made it beautiful or ugly, easy or hard. No longer was I a victim of circumstance, so self absorbed in my own misery that I missed the beauty and wonder of each unfolding day. Like Atlas, the weight of the world had been lifted from my shoulders. By acting in the world through informed eyes, I'd still have to go about my own business, but I would be doing so with a lightness about my tasks. My perception would change the entire experience for me. By not placing judgement on the events and people I came in contact with, I, in essence, freed myself to experience the moment as a fully realized soul. I programmed my brain to perceive the beauty and simplicity of life instead of its misery.

Your brain functions much the same way as a computer. It houses your thoughts, beliefs and perceptions. Information comes into the brain through your senses. It is unlike the sense of intuition that is a different kind of knowing that comes from the Universal Mind and is received all at once. Physical senses give you splintered information. The brain then gathers the information, firing the synapses with trillions of these bits until it recalls some type of wholeness based upon a past experience. Your personality self then interprets this information into memory, learning, dreaming, imagining, coordinating, controlling or decision making. The brain does not qualify this information, your personality does. The brain acting like a computer takes in the information (your perception of a stimulus) and stores it into the computer (your mind or the sum total of all experiences, judgements and beliefs). Your mind then qualifies it, for example, "I can't stand this relationship anymore," or

"I hate my job," or "I hate myself for doing that." Your brain has about 10 billion association neurons and yet you only use a portion of this immense capacity. The brain is goal seeking and problem solving. That is all it does twentyfour hours a day seven days a week except during extremely stressful situations when it takes a short break. If you are not constantly in the growing mode (creating or reaching a goal), the brain will create a problem. So the trick is to give the brain something to work on—short term and long term.

Because the brain is literal, amenable to suggestion, non controversial, cannot tell the difference between what is real and imagined and has no sense of humor, it is easy to program. You can program your brain to help you reach your goals. If you need a new car, new house, new job, new partner, or a new self image, put it into your computer. To program your brain, you need to get quiet. No distractions. Use plenty of juice, emotional juice, (let yourself get emotional) to electrochemically fire new synapses in the brain. That imprints the message into your being. This should give you a clue as to why certain behaviors are so hard to change. Once a synapse is created, it remains there forever. You cannot erase a synapse (dissolve an old belief). You need to create a stronger, more powerful new synapse (belief) which will eventually dominate the old belief. Your new beliefs associated with your new actions will strengthen your new behavior, until the new belief system becomes fully incorporated into your being by your focused energy. Can any of you remember when as a child, you touched something hot and got burned? Hot! Pain! Tears! You created a synapse in your brain that was so powerful, you probably never again touched that thing.

The brain works by creating synapses all the time. It is a tool for you to use in your everyday life. Creating new patterns for yourself can cut to the core of a problem. Let's say you constantly criticize yourself for being overweight as my former patient did. By adding fuel to that belief with self criticism and guilt, you put the focus in the wrong place. Maybe the original synapse was created by a parent's comment during your chubby phase as an infant. Because you bought into what your parents told you about yourself, your life style now perpetuates or supports that belief in all four of your natures. Because of possible dysfunctional relationships with parents, family or friends, you added more distance (fat) between yourself and the external world. Since your brain will not allow you to grow past the image of yourself you must first change your self image. At this point you find yourself easily losing weight by changing a life long pattern.

To reprogram your self image, close your eyes and see your face in front of you as if you were looking into a mirror. Notice your hair as it falls on your forehead and the shape of your face. If you have trouble doing this, look into a mirror and open and shut your eyes several times until you can see your face with your eyes shut. Look into your eyes, the windows to your soul, and see a child that is curious, playful, and fun to be with. Now see self confidence and wisdom. See a glow surrounding your face, the glow of beauty, harmony and intelligence. This is love surrounding you. Notice a smile crossing your lips which is joy bubbling up from within. Feel the joy of knowing that you have the courage to change and that you are worthy to receive all the good in the Universe. Do this selfimaging program twice a day and your brain will form a new synapse. Look at yourself often in the mirror and say your full name as it appears on your birth certificate. Your name, or logos, is your calling card to communicating with your higher self and connecting with your purpose here on Earth.

Your ego is located at the base of your neck. Its function is to screen out beliefs that do not fit into your current belief system. Because the brain is literal and noncontroversial it will accept whatever information is fed into it as fact. Therefore, it is important to become aware of what is being fed into your computer. Being amenable to suggestions means putting in the right input (a pleasant thought) that can literally change the entire experience for you. What you feed into your conscious and unconscious mind is as important as what you feed your physical body. If, for example, you are always telling yourself "give me a break," you may end up with a fractured femur. You must become as aware of your mental diet as you are of your nutritional diet. Are you being influenced by the belief systems of those around you? How are you influenced by advertising, education, government, media, religious leaders and family or friends? Since thought directs energy, whatever you focus on will grow. If you focus on the goal of going Home, you will go Home; focus on your problems and your problems will grow.

Affirmations can be a very sustaining part of your mental diet. One useful affirmation to say are the words, "I am now evolving mentally, physically, emotionally and spiritually. My path is being opened before me and I am now going down it. Thank you guys (God, guides, counselors, upper management) for all of your help."

Have you ever noticed that once you gain some insight into why you have been performing some destructive behavioral pattern, you can usually release it from your life? It's as if at some higher level you made the decision to change, and your ego allowed the information to come through. Counselors, physicians, priests, ministers or best friends can help you become aware of destructive patterns. If you need to talk about your problem, find someone you feel comfortable with and do so. When you get the Aha! do something about it. If you do not want to do what it takes to change then do not keep feeding your problem by talking about it. Similarly, if you are the listener, do not keep listening to someone with the same old problem. They like their problem.

Often your ego will block you from gaining insight into a particular situation. If this happens, program your brain to bring the information to you a different way. I (Peter), remember telling someone who could not get to an Aha! about a situation, to keep track of their dreams. When the ego puts up a defense in the conscious mind, the dream says, "No problem. I'll draw you a picture." Dreams give you a direct link to the subconscious mind, and to your night life. Dreams can be either literal, lucid, or they can be symbolic. Depending on how much time you sleep, you spend approximately one third of your life dreaming. This is an untapped wealth of information for you. Almost everyone and everything you dream about in a symbolic dream is about yourself, although the characters and the situations don't appear to be you.

If you dream you fall off a ladder, the first thing you should ask yourself is, "was the dream literal?" If you planned on fixing your roof the next day, you may want to check the rungs on the ladder. If they're okay, then what was the symbolism behind the dream? Do you reach your goals only halfway? What if one night you find yourself dreaming that you're out in the middle of an ocean and you're drowning— no help in sight? Unless you are about to take a cruise, where in your life are you drowning?

Dreams are real. People have died in their sleep while dreaming. If you find yourself in an anxious or frightening dream wake yourself up. Then change the experience to some thing positive. Working with your dream can change your waking life. You find yourself walking down a heavily wooded path. It's dark. The air is thick and heavy with stillness. You're finding it hard to breathe. You hear some sort of an animal ahead of you. Your heart starts pounding. You are now gasping for air. A huge Bengal tiger slinks around a bend in the path. You know you are his dinner. You wake up in a sweat, palms clammy, heart pounding off your chest. Get up and go to the bathroom. Pour yourself some water. Do whatever it takes to calm yourself. Then go back to the point in the dream when you started to get emotional and recreate that moment. Face the tiger but this time open the path up into a grassy meadow. Bring in sunlight and a calm breeze. Now turn the tiger into a big pussycat that comes loping through the meadow to greet you. You open your arms wide, and the weight of him knocks you down while he licks your face. You roll with him and scratch his ears and belly. You are so happy to see each other. You have changed your perception and therefore your emotional response. You have just taken care of some business. This will translate into your daily life. It may be a new client you will meet in a couple of days or something from the past that was still hunting you.

There are four universal symbols that may help you interpret your dreams: fire represents change, purification and transformation. Air represents spirit, thoughts. Water represents emotions and Earth represents the material world. What if you cannot remember your dreams? Program your brain at night to remember them. Simply inhale deeply while you inhale roll your eyes upward into the back of your head. Then exhale and allow your eyes to roll forward. This immediately puts you into an Alpha state, which means your brain is ready to be programmed. Put in whatever you want. It would be a good idea to tell your computer that you want to be with your teachers and you want to remember all your dreams and wake up feeling rested and peaceful. You can add to that a physical sensation. Drink a couple of tall glasses of water right before you go to bed. You should get up sometime in the middle of the night and catch one of those dreams on your way to the bathroom.

And if you still can not remember your dreams, you can get a sense of their emotional nature: fear, joy, sensual, freeing, etc. If you find yourself in the middle of a sexual dream, enjoy it and do not feel guilty when you wake up. The ultimate goal is to be lucid and in control during your dream state and functioning from your mental body during your awake and sleep states, remaining connected to spirit at all times. In this manner you will be well into your goal of al-ways functioning from spirit.

CHAPTER 5
SPIRITUAL WELLNESS

As you bring into harmony your physical, emotional and mental bodies, you are ready to move more fluidly into the capstone of all bodies: the spiritual body. This is the body that vibrates at the highest frequency. The God soul resides in this important body and represents a direct link between you and the Creator. The goal of every incarnate soul is to function from this level at all times. To get there requires a great deal of commitment, dedication and humility. You must completely dissolve the ego. Obviously this is no small task; in fact, some will say it is almost an impossible task to achieve. That is the key question. Is it possible for a human to achieve this level of consciousness in a single lifetime? And if so, what happens to the other bodies, in particular to the physical body, when this exalted state, referred to as Christ Consciousness, God-Realization or Home is reached? Another question to ask is, "How does one get there?" Many more souls than just Christ and Buddha have gone before you and were able to reach this level of consciousness. They accomplished this formidable task and in so doing have opened the doors for you, to let you know it is indeed possible to obtain GodRealization. No doubt it is difficult, as is any goal worth dedicating oneself to, but it is possible!

Once you have reached this goal and transmuted your consciousness, the other bodies will be pulled in one by one, down to and including the physical body, to begin resonating at the same exalted state. Transmutation of the physical body begins by reaching a level of consciousness made possible by maintaining Karmic neutrality. Void of Karma you then move to a higher level of awareness, not ruled by the ego, which allows greater Light to enter your body by way of the chakras. At this point the Divine energy is transmitted to every atom in your body, instantly changing its vibrational frequency to begin resonating at the Christ frequency level. In this manner you merge with God's consciousness and achieve, among other things, eternal life. Interesting concept, but is it true? Can you actually change every cell in your body to make a new body, a so called "light body?" How do you know you have successfully achieved transmutation? As one of our teachers told us several years ago when we asked that question, "You know because you got there." Admittedly, these are profound questions that go beyond everyday life circumstances, yet everyone on the planet should be working toward this attainable goal. The trick is to translate these lofty ideas into everyday life. To help you unravel the mystery I (Peter), will reveal a personal incident that took place several years ago which illustrates how to work through a difficult situation, learn from the experience and move forward toward the goal of spiritual wellness. One crisp summer morning I took my notepad and sat on the beach to write this chapter, but the information simply would not come. Shortage of natural beauty certainly could not account for my lack of inspiration, since Captiva Island has one of the most beautiful shorelines in the country. Having learned by that point that it is best not to force things, I put my pen away and decided to enjoy the beach instead. Several days later the inspiration finally arrived bright and early at 5:00 A.M. on a Thursday morning. Thursdays used to be the busiest day of my week because I would see patients in the office and do all my surgical cases as well. That morning started differently. My wife had been staying at our cottage in Captiva that was about 300 miles from our home in Orlando. On this morning I was to leave after my morning office appointments to join her. I hoped to get more writing done but the Universe had other plans for me.

I woke up at 5:00 A.M. and began my daily ritual asking God to guide me through my daily activities, to help me to remain spiritually connected and to help me see and understand all the signs that would be placed along my path. Another way of saying this is to grant me the gift of sight and sound as situations unfold and opportunities for spiritual growth present themselves. Once out of bed I went into the bathroom. Suddenly I heard a loud noise that sounded like a rainstorm coming out of the main closet. I opened the door to the closet and to my amazement boiling water was pouring out of the ceiling, all over our clothes and everywhere. I immediately climbed up to the attic to investigate and discovered the hot water heater tank, which was mounted on top of the closet, had burst and hot water was gushing out soaking the insulation, electrical wiring and ceiling. A great big lake had formed on the sheet rock above the closet and the pressure was about to give way. God, why did this happen? Water, I concluded, means emotions. Hot water, hot emotions. Anger? Am I angry with someone or something? Is someone going to be angry with me later in the day? Is the house angry because Elizabeth and I have decided to move west?

First things first. I climbed down from the attic and quickly called the man who had just installed another expensive component to our incredibly complicated water purification system. He suggested I shut off the water valve to the tank. Good idea! As soon as I did that the flood stopped and I could think more clearly. As I was driving to the hospital for a 7:30 A.M. case, I kept asking why? Why did this "accident" happen? I asked the Universe for help in deciphering what I was supposed to learn from this unpleasant experience. Remember, the Universe is feminine in nature and therefore hidden from you. It works through symbols, so to appreciate your lessons, you must learn to interpret the symbolic meaning of situations that present themselves. In this manner you evolve through the spiritual lessons that are being presented rather than reacting to situations with emotional discord.

As one learns to make this connection on a daily basis, the opportunity to learn from the experience and heal a part of yourself is made possible. In my own situation, by the time I drove into the parking lot at the hospital (approximately thirty minutes away) I had an answer. The "accident" was meant for me; after all, I was the only one in the house. The hot water represented an outpouring of hot emotions I had experienced the night before upon learning that my wife had a newly discovered male friend on the Island. When she first told me about this man in great excitement, I had become jealous that he had befriended my partner. Her interest in him was due to her discovery of his knowledge about yinyang principles concerning the balancing of energies. I realized that part of the belief system I was raised with was that friendships between men and women were not permitted. This dramatic incident was a gift that enabled me to examine an incorrect belief system that had enslaved my life. This theme of emotional outpouring was to resurface later in the day.

I quickly released my jealousy and instead thanked the Universe for this man's friendship to my wife and subsequently to myself as well. I completed the surgery uneventfully and decided to call our builder for advice. The house was less than a year old, so I felt the water heater would probably still be under warranty. The phone call gave us an opportunity to heal some old wounds that had developed during the construction phase of the house. I had forgotten all about them, but apparently he had not. I was genuinely glad to hear his voice again and to have the opportunity to put closure on past issues. After a few minutes he decided to help us in whatever way he could and later the phone rang with the news that the plumber was on his way. Great news!

The office was slow. One new patient had canceled and I found myself with extra time to see an "old" patient. She was a rather attractive thirty year old whom I had not seen in two years. Mary had come in requesting birth control pills but also complained of a painful vaginal opening. She seemed unusually nervous during the examination. When the nurse left the room she said to me "I didn't want to say anything in front of your nurse but. . .I haven't told you the truth." At that point she burst into tears and still smiling said "I have no money. I'm now on my own. . .I had no choice." I asked her what she meant and she replied "Well, I'm a working girl." I then asked "Do you mean you are prostituting yourself?" "Yes," she yelled out and started crying again.

She went on for a while to tell me about all the terrible things that were around her and how she felt totally out of control. I just sat and listened to the purging of emotions in a way I had not seen anyone else do in twelve years of private practice.

Just like my water heater tank, she was outpouring feelings of despair and anger about herself. As she spoke, I felt a chill right up my spine and realized it had been no coincidence that all events of the day led to this point. I knew I was supposed to listen carefully to every word she said and then plant a seed for her needy soul.

After she was through, I went on to advise her in the best way I knew how, which was to stress her need to empower herself and to stop looking for the answers to her predicament outside herself. By reinforcing the necessity to begin the healing process from within, life would then offer her other choices not presently seen. My comments seemed to console her, although she was obviously still shaken by the emotional episode. Only time will tell if the seed I planted in her mind will grow. I feel that it will since our meeting was arranged for a higher purpose.

As you read about my experiences some of you may conclude that, although the specific details of the episode were unique to me and my patient, situations such as the one I described happen to people every day. Perhaps they have even happened to you. Whereas most individuals would have reacted in anger to the morning "accident" with the water heater, the fact that I chose not to and instead saw it as a sign from the Universe made all the difference in the world to me and my patient. Not only did the Universe provide a wonderful opportunity, albeit dramatic, for me to learn a lesson, but it also left me clear headed to advise my patient in a caring manner untainted by my own discomfort. What a great way to inspire the writing of a chapter on spiritual wellness! What a wonderful illustration to show me the spirituality of all things.

Everything is spiritual. Everything in the manifested Universe is provided for you and all living beings for the purpose of unfolding the spirit. Everything was created for the spirit to appreciate the connectiveness of all events, no matter how remote and insignificant they may seem to you. It is only because of an individual's limited consciousness that s/he often fails to make the connection and appreciate the higher purpose of what happens to him/her. You must remember there is a Higher Will and a greater plan which you are part of. There is also a hierarchy and everybody has a "boss!" A crucial step is to surrender yourself to God.

Humility is one of the first requirements of the initiate as s/he embarks upon his/ her journey Homeward. How can someone who thinks s/he knows it all ever learn something new? You must be willing to humble yourself be-fore God. Part of this surrendering process is to release your preconceived beliefs about life and open yourself to new possibilities, new ways of seeing things.

To set the record straight let me say that in Cosmic terms, all the accumulated knowledge humans have mastered since the beginning of time can be placed on the sharp end of an ordinary pin. Now. . . does that make you feel better about yourself? Do you still think you have great wisdom? I certainly do not, and yet, I love and respect myself for what I do know about life. As my faith grows, I increase my awareness and knowledge of God. Faith is a difficult concept for many people to accept; believing there is a God, a Divine Plan for the daily events that unfold along your path is sometimes difficult to accept. As a child I (Peter), was taught to believe in God; as a teenager I struggled to keep faith in God and now as an adult I have learned that faith opens doors. Beyond faith comes knowing. This knowingness is the understanding that the Creator always was, is and shall always be a part of me. This knowingness came about developmentally, intuitively and through the integration of love into everyday mundane activities.

A few years ago we felt compelled to move West and, to our amazement, in less than forty days we were able to close our practice, sell our office building, and sublease our cottage in Captiva. Countless incredible events took place over the next nine months that culminated in a totally new life direction for both of us as we became fully committed to our spiritual growth and to being of service to others. You must let go of the old to make room for the new, but while you are between shores, it is faith that carries you.

Understanding the fundamental truth that a soul will attract to itself what it needs to experience places the seeker in a powerful position to become aware of his/her actions on a moment to moment basis. As you proceed along your path, you transform yourself into a light beacon and attract others into your energy field. Service becomes a way of life as you evolve to higher levels of consciousness. Christ said "I am here to share a knowledge of things with you and also to serve you. " His words symbolize your innate ability to give and receive love. Being of service to others can be done in many different ways. Part of my service to humanity is the writing of this book which I hope will present an alternative voice to the mounting cries of fear, anger and separateness from God. Helping individuals like the patient I described earlier to see that true power is within is part of my service. Yours may be holding a frightened child's hand, visiting an elderly person, or perhaps giving a few words of encouragement to another soul while waiting for a bus. As you serve others, you also serve yourself by evolving spiritually. By being there 100% and listening to my patient's call, I received the gift of hearing my own words saying to her: look inside yourself for all the answers concerning your soul. As you begin to see the Godaspect of everything, mundane activities take on new meaning. Breathing, for example, becomes the ability to take life-force or prana into your being. Eating and drinking, symbolizing physical nourishment of your temple from Mother Earth and the hands of those who prepare the meals including your own. This is another expression of receiving love from others. Sleeping is seen as quiet time: an opportunity to meditate and be with God and gain glimpses of your innerself through the dream state unfiltered by the personalityself or ego, a chance to visit other realities. Communicating with others (humans, animals and plants) is interpreted as exchanging love and thought forms, hopefully of an uplifting nature. Exercising your physical body is seen as an activity to integrate your spirituality into your body and maintain a balance in all four aspects of your being (spiritual, physical, mental and emotional). All activities taken as a whole thus represent opportunities to learn lessons and a way to escape the Wheel of Karma and return to the Oneness from whence you came.

How lonely, how desperate, how full of suffering life must be to those who have either forgotten or have denied they are creatures of God! An illustration of this misconception is the patient described earlier who felt lost and disconnected from the world around her. In contrast, there are countless souls who wander around life thinking and believing they have all the answers. The answer to the mystery of life is not out there but inside you. Loving yourself as a complete, fully integrated, pure and perfect spiritual being starts the process of self healing and receiving Grace from God. You are God manifested. Every cell in your body carries all the wisdom of the Universe, since everything is connected to everything else. I often used to ask myself the question: "Who is God?" The question I now ask myself is, "Can anything exist that is not God?" You are all part of a giant matrix which is called God.

For those who doubt the existence of God I would ask a few questions: Has anything ever happened to you that you could not explain based on your current belief system? For instance, did you ever see a lighter physical form or so called spirit? Did you hear something unexplainable such as voices or the sound of violins or bells?

Have you ever had an out of body experience? Did you ever have a premonition about an event that was later confirmed to be true? I am certain most of you answered yes to at least one of those questions. Those of you who have no recollection of ever having an extraordinary experience most likely dismissed the episode as your imagination playing tricks on you. You are conditioned by society to extend the limits of your consciousness to your five physical senses. To most people such momentary expanded states of consciousness are attributed to overwork, stress, or nervous disorders. You are quick to rationalize such events and find a physical explanation for their occurrence, fearing ridicule from others or worse still: madness. Presently most Western societal institutions do not support such levels of awareness.

Another question I may ask from those of you who still refuse to believe in Divine Guidance is this: Have you ever experienced a time in your life when everything seemed to go wrong? Conversely, how about another period of your life when ordinary events flowed effortlessly. Now for the sake of argument, accept the existence of a Divine Plan and agree that God is undeniably real. Reexamining both sets of conditions previously mentioned as opportunities given to you to unfold

In spirit, isn't it easier to appreciate the value of those experiences when seen as lessons? It is because of your belief systems that you learn to judge events as good or bad. The emotional response is largely based on what the intellect or ego chooses to integrate into the personality self.

In my life the water heater incident could have been inter preted as a negative experience. Yet, when studied from a higher perspective, it became an extremely important sign to resolve some personal issues that were impeding my spiritual growth. Pleasant experiences can also be lessons that aid in your spiritual unfoldment. Being able to identify repeating behavioral patterns that signal something is not flowing is the Universe's way of communicating with you. If you are accident prone and keep hurting yourself, it is useful to ask yourself this question: Why am I constantly hurting myself? Why am I punishing myself? Accepting the existence of God not only helps explain life events but also serves as nourishment in realizing you are not alone. Even the word gives you a clue as to what it really means: ALLONE.

When you learn to appreciate the Godliness of all things, seeing the beauty and harmony of nature untouched by humankind becomes a part of you. You feel connected to everything in a way that explains your human condition as an integral part of a larger reality that includes all things on Earth and in the heavens. You begin to understand how your body works much like a small scale cosmos with many similarities to the solar system. Just as there is harmony in the heavens, so too are you meant to have harmony within yourself. Scientists continue to discover new forces that explain the behavior of solar bodies. Einstein, for example, was also working on a single theory to explain how the Universe works. Spiritually this is what we call connectiveness. In other words, what is true of a sub particle must also be true of a constellation.

I used to feel confused by such expansive concepts, not fully understanding mathematically what I sensed spiritually. I now realize spiritual laws are no different than physical laws except one must accept the idea of other realities existing beyond the three dimensional "real world" you and I share in this Universe. As humans we are taught to place most of our focus on this denser physical world, which is why traveling faster than the speed of light seems impossible. Time does not exist in other realms of existence, therefore speed is not a major consideration.

Thought directs energy. You move your consciousness by a mere thought. An instant later you are there. Spiritual evolvement ultimately leads the individual to learn ways to transfer his/her consciousness to other realities. Outofbody experiences are but one example of this innate ability all humans possess. The human can travel to different levels of consciousness or degrees of awareness as the individual learns to evolve spiritually.

I recall the first time I experienced a willed outofbody experience. I was working in a small town in South Carolina and brought with me a book on the subject. One afternoon I decided I was ready to willfully separate my spirit from my physical body and thus, with some apprehension, I began to meditate focusing on this goal. Several hours later I was still in bed with my face facing North and nothing happening. I opened my eyes and realized fear of death was keeping me from succeeding. This time I decided to release the fear that was holding me back and do my best to achieve the goal. I closed my eyes again in meditation and a few moments later I began to lift away from my physical body. As I began to separate I could feel my own breath behind the back of my head. In excitement I rotated my lighter body (astral body) and looked at myself (meat body) resting peacefully. At this point I could not rightfully describe in words the feeling of elation I experienced! I immediately decided to explore and in a matter of a few seconds I found myself being taken to another reality. I recall a female voice saying to me "Peter, now and again we will take you to different places."

I landed in a square where a multitude of souls were feasting on ice cream, riding on rides and having a great time. Everyone I met was extremely loving and kind. I remember asking myself, "do these souls know I come from planet Earth?" After a while I was brought back and as I returned I thanked my teachers (guides) for the unforgettable experience. I spent the next few days trying to repeat the experience to no avail. I finally decided that mastering separation from the physical body was not my goal, but that transmutation and service as a

Multiverse (Multiple Universes) citizen was. One of the many benefits this trip had for me was to prove that humans can travel to other realities or Universes. This experience also removed all fear of death by confirming to me, beyond the shadow of a doubt, that I was more than my physical body.

Often while dreaming or during meditation we visit other realities. The Hindu religion calls the dream state "little death." Fear of death is a major concern of most Westerners. How do you see death? Are you afraid of dying? In that last breath, will you be wondering whether you measured up to enter the Kingdom of Heaven? Or do you instead believe there is nothing beyond this life, only darkness? Before my first outofbody experience I too wondered what was on the other side. To me it did not seem to help to have faith. I did not believe that there had to be something else. Faith is different from knowing. I recall thinking of death and feeling my pulse rise, my breathing become shallower. Sometime later I had another outofbody experience that served to explain the mystery of death.

My father had passed away the year before and I felt I had not properly said goodbye to him. By the time I saw him at the hospital he was in and out of coma and unable to communicate with me. I recall the second outofbody experience took place the same day I decided to become a vegetarian and to stop drinking alcohol. I went to sleep as usual and woke up around five o'clock in the morning from an unpleasant dream. I got up and went to the bathroom and then went back to sleep.

This time I asked my teachers to help me see my father. A few moments later, and in full consciousness, I felt myself lifting out of my physical body. I then heard the rush of air through my ears as I traveled to another reality. I felt guided to a large beautiful building. I glided into a room in this building where I met a strikingly attractive Indian woman who handed me a gorgeous newborn. I picked up the baby and realized it was a girl. I then glided to another room that was brightly lit and there he was! My father, standing naked in front of me with a stethoscope around his neck staring back at me. (I felt the stethoscope symbolized his way of paying respects to my chosen profession in this lifetime). He looked much younger, about thirtyfive years old, and had his usual mustache. I immediately hugged him and then looked around noticing another girl about five years old and again the same woman I had seen earlier carrying the baby. I stood there for a while staring at all four of them and realizing I had been granted a wonderful gift: To be able to visit the soul who used to be my father, now married to a beautiful woman with two lovely daughters, saying goodbye to me for the last time. We looked at each other for a long time not saying a word and then I saw myself being pulled back into my physical body. I woke up and sat in bed and wept with my heart filled with joy and sadness at the same time. I was granted the rare privilege to visit my father in another world. Since then there have been more trips to other places. Each time it happens it is a confirmation to me, as I am certain it has been to those of you who have experienced similar extraordinary events, that there is no death. You simply go from one form to another. Our denser more compacted energy form changes to a lighter, faster energy form that allows us to travel to another dimension (Universe) where the time/space continuum does not exist. For me the whole experience has always been an uplifting one; in fact, I often feel a sense of disappointment upon my return to the physical world. I am certain many of you who have not had this kind of experience must wonder whether I am telling the truth or even if I'm crazy. After all, Western religious teachings do not support such states of consciousness.

It is important to understand that your consciousness may visit these levels based on your level of evolution and vibrational frequency. The Universe is comprised of five levels of vibrational frequency or distinctly different Universes. The lowest level is the physical realm. Next comes the Astral plane that has within itself several sublevels. As one transcends the levels, the vibration becomes more refined and one can travel at a faster speed. At the top end of the Astral level is what many Western religions describe as heaven. Likewise the lower region could be referred to as hell. Karma still exists at the Astral level and therefore the souls who reside there must eventually reincarnate to become karma free. A soul cannot move through karmic issues unless s/he has a body and can function in the physical world. Thoughts (desires) from the physical Universe feed the Astral Universe.

The next level or Universe is the Causal Plane that exists in a finer vibration. Human karma is completed at the lower portion of this plane. The fourth plane is called the Mental Plane that can only be visited or inhabited by souls that are karma free. Souls that are not karma free may not enter this level unless they are taken there by a teacher or guide. The final or fifth plane is called SAT NAM* (In Sanskrit meaning Truth be Its Name). This is the Universe we call Home, (also referred to as the 5th Dimension). It is a place where all souls eventually return. In the native American culture this is what is called the "Fifth Direction." It is filled with an incredible love, beyond all human understanding. Those who have achieved Godrealization are constantly operating from this exalted state. Your job is to learn to discern the subtleties in vibration of each Universe and to blend with those energies. The ultimate goal is to become so refined you function from spirit or SAT NAM (Truth Frequency) while being about your business in the physical world. Obviously only those individuals who have become karma free by doing their work can perform this feat.

Once the whole picture is understood, to the best of one's ability, it is easy to see why living an existence denying your spirituality is to function at a subhuman level not intended for the species. It is through the acceptance of yourself as a spiritual being that everything then becomes possible. You are God. You are spirit. You live in "one of the many orbs of God" called planet Earth. One of the greatest tasks on your spiritual journey is to overcome the three dimensional world of illusion or what Easterners call Maya, the physical world. Despite what you have been taught to believe, the material world is not reality, it is merely a reflection of spirit, which is the greater reality. Unfortunately, the opposite view has been drilled into people's minds, programmed only to accept what they can see, touch, smell, taste or hear. This distortion is precisely why you are so far removed from your spiritual nature. To understand spirit, in order to free yourself from the material world of illusion, you must cast your gaze toward the subtle world of spirit by turning inward. You must shut out the three dimensional world and go within. This is where you will find truth and peace. The world of illusion will fulfill you only momentarily, and after the newness of the experience has worn away, you are again hungry for another illusion to distract you. By contrast, the world of spirit will fulfill you completely because spirit is the true essence of the Universe. In the Western world when you hear of yogis who meditate for hours or live with very few material possessions you think them deprived, and that their lives are dull. This could not be farther from the truth. Riches of the soul come to those who can tune out the distractions of the physical world and go with in. Although the physical Universe was created for us to enjoy and learn more about ourselves, it should not take the center stage. Just as gold must be mined from deep within the bowels of the Earth, so are the riches of the spirit found deep within meditative states.

Section Three:

Dis- Ease and Modern Healthcare

A dis- eased society is like a cancer that eventually kills itself. Any health care System is doomed unless its beneficiaries become self-responsible individuals.

CHAPTER 6

DIS- EASE

What is the cause of dis- ease? Countless research institutions, prominent medical schools and Nobel prize winners have invested large amounts of time and money in this quest. Government and privately funded research continues to probe everything from the common cold to the rarest of all dis- eases. Every aspect of clinical medicine is undergoing scientific scrutiny to identify the cause of dis- ease. The simple fact is: All dis- ease, whether physical, emotional, mental or spiritual, is due to the misperception that you are separate from God. It's that simple. Always remember who you are and you will escape the plague of dis- ease. As you come to the realization you are God, the most infectious germ, deadliest environment or hazardous "accident," will have no hold on you. As you focus all your efforts on this goal, eventually your awareness will lead you to conclude that any scientific research without a spiritual foundation is superfluous.

The global scientific community is concentrating most of its resources on finding a cure for cancer, while completely ignoring the environment factors of increasing levels of toxicity from the 5G & Space X radiation, chem-trails and a multitude of other toxic environmental factors increasing daily. What is cancer? A cancerous cell can best be described as one with uncontrollable growth having total disregard for its neighboring cells. The dis- eased cell isolates itself while neglecting the needs of other cells to the detriment of the host. Similarly, when ruled by the ego, you go about life with total disregard for yourself, your fellow human and the environment, lacking the awareness that you too are part of a bigger picture called God.

You must get bigger than yourself. See yourself intricately connected to nature and those around you. Like the cancerous cell that disconnects itself from the whole of the physical body, so too do you disconnect from the wholeness of God. When your brain or intellect is running the show operating from a limited belief system, you are restricting the flow of Divine Principle from moving through every cell in your body. By focusing on your own selfish and petty demands rather than surrendering your will to God, you step on the hose thus cutting off the flow, and dis- ease strikes.

Imagine the Creator as a great Central Sun that radiates life giving energy much the same way our sun gives forth energy that supplies us with life. The energy from the great Central Sun is zillion times more powerful than our Sun. This energy is called Prana, Divine Principle or Holy Spirit. You are therefore the "Sun" of God receiving this holy spirit from the father, the Creator. This is the Holy Trinity. This Light from God comes into your physical body by way of chakras that are wheels of energy strategically placed throughout your body. As these energy vortices receive energy (Light) from the Creator, they begin to spin, emitting their own unique color and sound. This divine energy bathes each organ, tissue, and cell with radiating life, giving energy. The extent to which you are willing and able to receive this life giving energy is the extent to which you are dis- ease free. Your body is constantly being bathed by this Divine Principle that is powerful enough to give you complete sustenance without further need for the consumption of food, water, or air if properly absorbed by your cells. The problem lies in your body's passage ways such as blood vessels and capillaries, lymphatic system, respiratory and intestinal tract, becoming blocked with toxins and other impurities. As parts of your body become isolated from the rest by these blockages, dis- ease begins to set in.

This illustrates how separating your self from God and God's energy creates physical, emotional, mental or spiritual illness. These blockages can arise from a variety of different sources such as 5G wifi radiation, toxins and pesticides in the foods you eat, fatty deposits accumulated on the walls of your blood vessels, or excessive protein intake leading to kidney stones, arthritis, etc. Drugs and alcohol along with other harmful substances, have the same effect of blocking the flow of Divine Principle to every cell in your body. Emotional and mental toxins can also block this flow of spirit through your body. Holding on to old hurts and blames and traumas, adopting beliefs that encourage a low self esteem support separation from God. This will block the flow of this holy and healing energy and lead to emotional or mental illness. Feeling fearful, angry, sorrowful or unworthy all limit your ability to bathe and nurture yourself with the radiance of the Divine Principle.

Your soul's complete unfoldment can be thought of as a continuum or composite of all your previous lifetimes leading up to the present. Unfortunately, few have recall of previous life experiences and thus, even as children, it is easy to repeat mistakes from the past that keep you trapped in the Wheel of Karma. Consider a soul who returns to Earth following a lifetime exemplified by theft and violence. As a child this person may be seen taking toys from other children, stealing small change from their mother's purse or physically abusing a younger brother or sister. As this individual enters adulthood, the mischievous activities from his/her childhood assume a more serious social connotation repeating the same patterns seen in an earlier life. If the individual comes to a higher level of awareness, the opportunity to reach karmic neutrality can begin. Perhaps this opportunity will take the shape of serving humanity as a social worker, counselor or another profession that allows the individual an opportunity to repay his/her karmic debt. In some way the cosmic doors will open so that s/he may repay his/her debts. This system also explains why certain individuals are born with birth defects or physical/mental impairments that would be labeled senseless if the explanation were solely confined to a single lifetime. The sight of a malnourished infant born to a mother in the Sudan, hopelessly breast feeding, may invoke pity but it should be regarded as remedial reading for that soul, since these are conditions that help the individual work through karmic debts. Therefore there is no need to feel sorry for these souls who will return in a better position next time around. Granted, on the surface, it may be difficult to rationalize why a baby is born to live only a few hours or is even born dead, has any value. The parents, who are left devastated by such a calamity, may find it extremely difficult to accept the redeeming value of such an experience.

Nevertheless, these and other similar events labeled as unfortunate are all part of a Divine Plan. Accepting with faith the lessons that are presented to you can often be a test of courage and commitment to your spiritual path. The same principle applies to a soul choosing his/her biological parents as the best environment in which to fulfill his/her life purpose and to complete the required course work. To see this connection one must look beyond the personalities of each parent and identify specific behavioral characteristics in the chosen parents that will likely be incorporated into one's persona. You may have chosen an alcoholic father and a submissive mother only to bring into focus your pattern of submissive behavior.

Look at every belief you have acquired since birth to the present and decide whether it is still valid for you. As you examine each belief ask yourself if it is bringing you closer to the Creator and perfect health. A religious belief that can hinder an individual's spiritual growth leading to dis- ease is the concept of "original sin." This is a disability that over one billion souls are born into across the planet. Over the course of many years, for some a lifetime, this message is repeated adnauseam, branding the individual as unclean and imperfect because of a symbolic event, which took place eons ago. Yet the Christian world believes one is still unforgiven until one is baptized (purified from the original sin). For some individuals the psychological consequences of being branded as sinners can be quite serious as they learn to see themselves as dirty and their souls soiled. This internal criticism can be expressed by difficulties in the giving or receiving of love from self or others, an inability to live in abundance or lacking the capacity of self-forgiveness for an act committed long ago. This religious belief is saying that something is wrong with you. The internal struggle that results as the individual constantly punishes him or herself for being a sinner continues until a serious mental or physical illness is manifested as the price paid for his/her perceived short comings (sins).

Most dis- ease can be linked to feelings of guilt in one form or another. Other life stresses can similarly manifest as illness unless the individual is constantly aware of his/her own unique path. For example, some parents criticize negative qualities in their children's personality in a misguided attempt to encourage them to succeed. Frequently this sets the tone within the individual's mind that s/he is bad, unworthy and shameful. A pattern is then established where criticism is the rule insteadof positive reinforcement. Most often this is done with the best of intentions to motivate the individual to improve on his/her shortcomings (as judged by the parents). Unfortunately, the message heard by the young soul's small and impressionable ears is that s/he is a bad person. From the parent's perspective their child is falling short of some goal they could not reach themselves but expect their child to accomplish. Within the child the feeling of unworthiness becomes a permanent aspect of his/her personality, thus the child learns to see himself/her self as unfit or unworthy to receive love from self or others. This creates more stress that begins to filter itself through the young body with visible results such as learning disabilities and/or behavioral disorders manifested in those who cannot take the constant pressure.

Sibling rivalry is another stressful situation. By having to constantly prove your worthiness to your parents who seem to favor a brother or sister, you are placed under constant pressure to perform. Nightmares, arguments with siblings and/or illnesses are unnatural states created by individuals to win the love and approval from parents. Fear of abandonment is ever present in the mind of a little person whose entire existence is dependent upon a big person. These little folks want so much to be loved and accepted, but when the parent is unable to give properly balanced love, the child feels that there is something wrong with him/her. While trying to please their parents, many children stop moving to their own unique rhythm, giving up their own true nature to become what they imagine their parents want them to be. Once they move away from their own rhythm, they become unbalanced and leave themselves open for a dis- ease to strike. It is important to remember children are complete human beings, they are just short! As the individual grows up and begins schooling, another set of conditions emerge that in addition tests ones ability to remain self centered and self assured while developing self esteem. School and athletics take on a competitive nature as students struggle to make the grade or the team as the case may be. School becomes an arena where competition prevails in all social activities. In most learning institutions, winning becomes the ultimate goal. Aggressive behavior is glorified over human kindness and cooperation. Personal growth takes a back seat to learning ways to beat the opponent or make the grade. Proving you are better than your adversaries justifies almost any kind of social behavior imaginable as long as you come out on top. Testing your worthiness by either becoming a winner or looser only serves to set up an egotistical dysfunctional social pattern which eventually leads one to the wrong conclusion that they are better than others or conversely the belief that they are a failures when compared to others. The emphasis on competing is carried on throughout life affecting many other areas.

As schooling is completed and the individual enters the workplace, competition is again placed at the highest level of importance. The fruits of your craft are compared to those of your rival, pitting you against another in competition. The emphasis is placed on an external goal (how well others like your work) rather than the internal goal of completing a task to the best of your ability and what you are learning about yourself in the process. Thus, one is deprived of self discovery and the satisfaction of a job well done.

I (Peter), treated a patient in a small Midwestern community. Frances came to the office concerned about a long battle with depression that she thought might be related to a hormonal imbalance. The clinical history revealed she had a very low self esteem regarding her obesity. A life long pattern of overeating followed every major conflict she ever had. This became a vicious cycle that perpetuated itself as she saw herself become fatter and fatter. After years of self inflicted physical abuse she sought the help of several psychiatrists and psychologists who placed her on numerous mood altering medications. She heard I practiced holistic medicine and decided to give me a try. Her obvious problem was her obesity (close to 250 pounds and five feet four inches tall) and a mildly elevated blood pressure.

I informed her that the depression was not related to a hormonal imbalance, although one did exist due to her obesity, which interfered with ovulation. Consequently an estrogen build up existed in her body that led to fluid retention that manifested as obesity. She responded "Yeah, other docs have told me the same thing but I don't know what to do." I could tell by her reaction to my questions she still refused to make a connection between her physical appearance (obesity), and the emotional dis- ease (low self esteem and depression) which had followed her most of her adult life. The nutritional history revealed a fat rich, flesh rich diet with no exercise.

My advice to her consisted of pointing out how often individuals internalize conflicts that can lead to a number of dis- eases and stressing the need for her to start the process of healing from within. By starting with a program based on improving her self image, she could wean herself off the medications and start a healthy diet and an exercise program. I informed her that the key to a successful treatment plan depended upon how much she could empower herself to regain a sense of self confidence and self worth. I stressed the fact that self love and spiritual centeredness would reveal themselves as new attributes in her personality as she learned to visualize herself as thinner, attractive, childlike and full of wisdom. Although I was called to another assignment a few weeks later, I felt some of the seeds I planted may have taken root. Perhaps for the first time in her life, she felt she could take charge. My job was done.

As this patient illustrates, it is easy to get caught in a wave of self criticism that will eventually manifest as a dis- eased state in your body. Modern life is full of traps and belief systems that bombard the individual with stressful situations. It is crucial to remember that true strength comes from within yourself, thus setting you free from the expectations of others and consequently allowing one to remain calm, centered and less likely to allow dis- ease to filter in. Instead of following someone else's agenda, learn to follow your own. Repeatedly one receives the message that they are unworthy, sinful, unlovable or shameful from school, work, religion and family. Is it any wonder dis- ease is so prevalent in today's society? You don't have to look far to see that we are doing it wrong. It is time to start on a new path towards wholeness and dis- ease free living.

Often when you begin to move out of old patterns, physical and emotional turmoil in the form of a Healing Crisis may follow, as you struggle to overcome your current state. Often the act of throwing off toxins may result in a temporary state of discomfort but it is a necessary step in the process of purification. Not to worry.

You are simply cleaning house and the ill effects will soon pass. Remember, dis- ease manifests as you resist continuing down the spiritual path your soul has committed to.

Social dis- eases work on the same principle. By creating the illusion of separateness, a community, country or planet, will block the flow of Divine Principle that maintains a sense of cohesiveness and unity in all things. The social pain that follows this separation leads to disharmony and violence as certain groups of individuals begin to function with disregard (like the cancer cell) for the rest of the host (the community). As you can see, modern society tends to promote dis- ease, therefore, to reach wholeness, you must extract yourself from the throws of social consciousness and create your life anew, your own way. You are meant to function as a fully integrated physical, emotional, mental and spiritual being living a harmonious life with self and the environment and operating from intuition one hundred percent of the time.

When operating from a constant state of Godliness, you allow yourself the privilege of receiving all nurturing sustenance from the Divine Principle. Unhindered by dis- ease, every cell in your body will accept the fullest benefit from this divine force and the purification of all organs will begin. As toxins leave your physical, emotional, mental and spiritual bodies, a true state of harmony, balance and bliss will emerge, allowing you to be constantly nurtured and sustained by the Creator's Light. In this manner God's Light will illuminate all aspects of your being. Individuals who need the assistance of social health services to achieve a dis- ease free living state will only succeed in their goal by acting self responsibly through informed eyes and ears and working within the framework of social healthcare systems that promote self reliance and preventive medicine.

CHAPTER 7

MODERN HEALTH CARE & THE GLOBAL HEALTH CRISIS

Sometime in 1965 two twin programs were created in the U.S.. by the federal and state governments designed to pay for health services for senior citizens, the needy and the disabled. These programs were called Medicaid and Medicare. The original intent of the Medicaid program was to provide basic medical care for individuals who were in a temporary state of poverty and unable to purchase their own health insurance. By restoring physical wellness to these citizens, they could begin the process toward financial recovery. Unfortunately, I have seen countless examples of how the system fosters dependency, fails to meet the needs of its recipients and encourages irresponsible behavior. I will cite six different clinical scenarios that illustrate these points.

Two years ago I worked in a federally funded Indian Health Service hospital where I learned that only a fraction of the over all medical needs were being provided to the Native Americans. This sad state of affairs existed although medical assistance was part of this country's original bargain with them. In the hospital where I trained, prenatal care was prioritized to the detriment of non pregnant patients. A friend of mine, working as an internist in the same facility, recounted stories of essential services withheld due to inadequate funding and liberal dispersement of obstetrical care.

Another case demonstrates how Medicaid encourages irresponsible behavior. While in South Carolina, a patient who was thirty seven years old, unemployed, and bleeding heavily for months came to my clinic. After examining the patient I recommended a D&C. Almost embarrassed, she whispered that the Medicaid office had informed her recently she would not qualify for medical assistance unless she became pregnant. Ironically, in South Carolina only a few miles away is the remains of one of the largest Plantations in the South that housed over two thousand slaves. Today you can take a walking tour that is a narrated story of a young slave boy who died of an appendicitis because no doctor was called. Yet there was always care for the females giving birth since that increased the slave holder's wealth.

Another patient in the Midwest, who was on Medicaid elected to have a laparoscopic hysterectomy that would allow her to be discharged the next morning and go back to work in two weeks time. Sometime after her discharge from the hospital the administrator summoned me to his office to discuss her case. It seems the hospital billed Medicaid ten thousand dollars for their services and collected a total of five hundred dollars. I was astonished by his report. A traditional hysterectomy would have caused her considerably more pain and required a hospital stay of several days instead of twenty four hours. After six weeks the patient could resume work. But the hospital would have been compensated several thousand dollars more if I had performed the traditional hysterectomy.

In Arizona, a twenty seven year old patient with three children, came to my office requesting a tubal ligation. She had been separated from her husband for some time and as a single parent and head of a household, she immediately qualified for Medicaid. Under Medicaid rules the patient needed to wait a minimum of thirty days from the time she signed the consent form for sterilization before the surgery could be performed. To complicate matters, a pap smear that I took during her visit demonstrated a serious precancerous condition that needed immediate attention. The plan was to perform a biopsy of the cervix during the tubal ligation. As part of the preoperative laboratory work a pregnancy test was drawn, which showed she was eight weeks pregnant. At that point, under Medicaid rules, the surgery had to be canceled which made her quite angry and fearful because of the potential risk of leaving the cervical tissue unattended for another year. Although she accepted responsibility for her actions in conceiving another child when the marriage was ending, she did not possess the financial resources to terminate the pregnancy and therefore asked me to falsify the medical record to say she was having a miscarriage that would have qualified her for coverage. I refused her request and instead made a referral to another physician who would do the abortion for less than three hundred dollars. She still maintained her inability to raise the money, although she found a way to support a two pack a day cigarette habit.

These patients illustrate several points: First that the current medical system fails to meet the needs of its recipients and the system fails to make individuals responsible for their own health and actions but instead forces dependency upon others. It also illustrates that underlining agendas exist as to who receives healthcare and how it is delivered. The current Medicaid monster is costing the USA billions of dollars a year and has become a self serving institution that needs to be transformed into a social program that temporarily helps needy individuals evolve physically, emotionally, mentally, spiritually as well as financially and socially. The twin program, Medicare, was instituted to handle the needs of senior and disabled citizens in the nation. As Americans live longer, Medicare patients have grown in numbers. This has greatly affected the quality and accessibility of these essential services. What started out as a noble and humane idea has turned into a bureaucratic nightmare where administrative costs eat up more than half the funds collected in taxes, resulting in the neglect of millions of needy citizens who depend on those social programs for survival. Why is it that the Medicare system has become so inefficient? Is it because doctors have become greedy and have abused the program? Are healthcare facilities acting responsibly by demanding higher reimbursements for services being provided to government insured patients (seniors and the poor) to purchase expensive new technology? Is competition between hospitals and duplication of services affecting the national healthcare bill today? Or has there been a hidden agenda behind American Medicine that has laid the foundation for the policies implemented though the WHO (World Heath Organization) that have now affected the entire world?

Most other countries outside the USA have socialized medicine, but is socialized medicine doing its job? I (Elizabeth) have had several medical procedures performed in Italy. While living in Florence I was fortunate enough to go to a University Hospital of teaching a learning and received excellent surgical care for free. The Hospital stay certainly wasn't very conducive to healing but my life was saved. However in Sicily I saw the disastrous outcome of what socialize medicine has become. In a University hospital since the compensation of money was not there, many of the Doc's worked for noble motives such as teaching the young emerging physicians and took great pride in their work. But in Sicily, because there is no money the local people told me that most of the good Docs left. In fact even the Physicians there told me to leave Sicily for any major surgical procedures. There was however the element of caring which existed in the smaller towns but with the advent of C.O.V.I.D the hospitals quickly lost that. Families were not allowed to visit their loved ones and the wards became prisons where the staff was only compensated to administer "standard" C.O.V.I.D procedures and would receive three thousand euro when a patient died of C.O.V.I.D (a lot of money for a poor hospital.)

But are hospitals in the USA which have more money using their funds responsibly? Every hospital's dream is to become a famous medical center. Recently I was working in a small community with a small hospital. From what I could see the hospital was functioning quite efficiently and yet the Board of Directors had decided to build a totally new facility of a greater size across town. When I asked the administrator why they decided to spend millions of dollars to build a new hospital he answered, "One of the primary reasons was to attract more private patients who are currently leaving town to go to the nicer facility 25 miles away. Our marketing department told us that the new hospital will draw many of those patients back because we will look like a medical center, although the same faces will be seen in both places." His answer illustrates the mentality that prevails in most Private hospitals today, which is a competitive focus rather than a cooperative and united effort to curb the escalating healthcare costs.

Is this setting the foundation for the new techno medical trend placing the emphasis on consumerism to find a quick Cure for dis-ease by replacing dis- eased body parts with artificial ones. Or using biotechnology as the "cure all" for dis-ease. Are we creating a world where longevity and enhanced neural function is no longer our responsibility but bought and sold like a commodity? Are we creating a future, like what Dr. Sanchez, head of D.A.R.P.A's department of biotechnology predicted, a world of neurally enhanced haves and have nots? Are we making technology our God rather than the Divine Creator taking a short cut that may cost us our free will? This easy route to this "pseudo" healing is by eliminating the warning signs that spirit is no longer flowing with ease through the body and is out of sync with divine creation? Has Modern medicine found yet another way to mask our symptoms ignoring the predominate Disease of our world today living out of harmony with nature and our Mother Earth and the Creator? Are we being fast tracked to a future void of God, the natural rhythms of nature and our own inner divinity? Will we relinquish all responsibility for our own healing process. Will we choose to replace a diseased body part with technology instead of looking deeper into our physical, emotional, mental and spiritual pain and dis-ease to regain balance? Will we cease to be human?

And what will happen to the supposed "have nots"? Those who do not have the financial resources to pay for this "advanced" bio-techno medical world? Will the practice of eugenics become common place since hospitals now receive a higher compensation for the indigents who die rather than those they "save"? What kind of world will we be creating where the "haves" are dependent on technology for their very existence and those who can not afford the latest procedure are euthanized? What new race of humans are we creating? A race that is no longer humane? A race that has no compassion for their fellow human beings? A race of humans that have made technology their God and are dependent on technology for their very existence? Will medicine and the greed of its administrators and practitioners be responsible for ending the human race and bioengineering a new human void of compassion, creativity and a divine connection to the Creator? Will the human race passively play into this scenario by refusing to accept responsibility for their own health. By refusing to heal physically, emotionally, mentally and spiritually?

What about the Docs? Another factor affecting the definition of modern healthcare delivery systems concerns the area of consumer expectations. Are healthcare consumers acting responsibly by demanding the best medical services while taking absolution for the responsibility of their own health? Many attorneys are making a lucrative living by fueling the anger of patients who have experienced unfavorable outcomes. Are dissatisfied patients acting responsibly by suing doctors and hospitals every time there is a poor outcome? Is this forcing doctors to follow "standard" medical procedures for fear of being sued destroying the "Art of Medicine" and the use of their intuition? This lack of self responsibility for one's own healing has opened the door for the Medical system and now the legal system to take over the responsibility for the patients' health. This has paved the way for world governments to claim ownership of each human's body and created a climate conducive to the Medical Tyranny in which we now live. Many Docs have been forced by medical mandates to inject themselves and their patients with the corporate funded bio technology in order to continue to practice medicine over riding their Hippocratic oath of "Primum non nocere", "first do not harm". What karmic repercussions are they incurring by being part of this elaborate scheme and by not making patients responsible for their own health or being responsible for their own health? Already horrors about these "vaccinations" are beginning to surface and will continue in the years to come.

Society teaches most individuals, starting at an early age, to abuse their physical vehicles. This abuse can take the form of physical, mental, emotional and/or spiritual neglect. Physical abuse includes eating unhealthy foods, engaging in acts of anorexia and bulimia or pushing your physical body beyond its limits in competitive sports. This physical, mental and emotional abuse results from lack of self love. By holding onto old hurts and blames, stress then manifests as anxiety, depression or some other mental and/or physical disease. Spiritual emptiness leads people to seek fulfillment in alcohol or drugs that temporarily relieves the stress of an unbalanced lifestyle. The end result of any of these factors is serious and permanent harm to your physical body, ultimately debilitating the natural defenses that keep you healthy. As you grow old, these life long abuses begin to manifest as chronic and debilitating illnesses that contribute to maintaining the Healthcare budget in the stratosphere.

Now with the C.O.V.I.D. (Certification of Vaccination Identification Documentation) Crisis our Global Health system is being overtaxed with the over whelming task of taking care of an ever increasing population of dis-eased people who are experiencing the devastating effects of not properly healing themselves but only masking their deep underlying health issues combined with the devastating effects of poor diet, Big Pharm's bogus solutions of drugs and injections that are creating more harm in the long run all happening in a New World of ever increasing toxic 5G EMF waves and elevating radiation levels. But no one is allowed to discuss or even bring up these key environmental factors into the equation of our current global health crisis. These key environmental factors and the way they are interacting with those vaccinated as well as the effects those transmitting this biotechnology has is augmenting the already present disharmony in people's physical, mental, emotional, and spiritual natures now manifesting in their physical form. Because of all the above factors and the fact that our global medical community has been unable to properly diagnosis and treat the real cause of the dis-ease infecting the World's Population they have been rerouted to follow the "science" funded by private foundations created to support the World Health Organization's agenda of delivering a Vaccination as the "Cure All" for a "deadly" virus.

This bogus attempt to cure C.O.V.I.D. is blowing up in the face of the Medical Community as they observe the devastating effects of Modern Medicine's current attempts to restore balance to a dis-eased global society. The Karmic repercussions of individuals not accepting responsibility for their own health while living in an ever increasing toxic world in bodies that have numerous underlying health issues due to poor diet, unhealthy lifestyles, toxic environments and the refusal to look deeper into the dis-ease held within their emotional, mental and spiritual bodies is culminating in the perfect storm of a massive global health crisis.

Because of the medical community's limited training in Microbiology and bio-technologically this C.O.V.I.D. conspiracy is going to blow up in their face. For the Docs who still are humane this will result in feelings of futility and powerlessness as they struggle to help their ailing patients. When ordering a myriad of tests to properly diagnose the problem they will continuously draw a blank missing the forrest for the trees. Because in all their years of studying the "Science" the role of mitochondria as the building blocks of human health nor the effects of EMF waves on the health of mitochondria was never explained. They will be completely unprepared to meet the rising demands of the onslaught of dis-eased patients. They will be left helpless as more and more dis-eased patients flood the waiting rooms and emergency rooms. Those who remain within the system without changing it will have no choice but to succumb to the hospital's financial agenda where it is more profitable to kill the patient than cure them. While those serving a privileged clientele will usher in the New Era in Medicine where the elixir of life, the "cure all" for everything is Bio- technology or fusing man with machine and creating a new AI Saipan. Those who remain human-e who still have a thread of compassion and have the courage to seek answers outside the corrupted medical systems will become the New Co-healers of Earth. They will come together to help humanity reach a new balance leaving behind their dis-ease by first taking responsibility for their own health and then helping others to reclaim ownership and responsibility for their own bodily temple integrating and healing physically, emotionally, mentally and spiritually. Those healed, whole or holy ones will help humanity to fully align with the Bio rhythms of nature, our Mother Earth and the Creator restoring balance, harmony, unity and retuning to a lifestyle in harmony with the wisdom of our Ancient elders. This will give birth to a new organic Infinite human whose connection to the Creator will bring their organic divine technology online and they will not have to "buy" Artificial technology or be dependent on a finite external A.I. "hive" minded network for their cures, money, or power.

Another problem the medical community is facing is the fact that they do not understand the concept of a healing crisis, ascension mechanics or the affects the increasing organic electromagnetic energies coming from the sun and the photon belt have on the human body ie ascension symptoms. These elevated energies if not properly assimilated throughout the body will throw the body out of balance as it seeks a new alignment with the higher frequency of energies entering the body as it brings more light into it. As the cells are flooded with this increased light frequencies it displaces toxins and other miasma that is no longer able to survive in the higher light frequencies now absorbed into the cell. This often causes the underlying dis-ease held within the memories of the cells to surface as they exit the system. To the western medically trained practicer this looks like dis-ease and rather than allow or augment the purging of the toxins the medically trained eye whose focus is always on pathology will see this a something bad that must be stopped. They will recommend some course of action that halts the healing crisis and thus the body, mind or spirit is unable to release the toxic miasma and rebalance itself into a higher alignment of ease. This ultimately works against the patient causing the toxins to build up. The patient often becomes worse off. According to standard medical procedure the practitioner will either repeat the same procedures or do something more radical which many times results in augmenting the dis-ease or even death.

Even in the practice of alternative medicine many practicers take a similar approach as allopathic physicians only addressing the physical body. They prescribe herbal remedies, look at diet, use energy modalities never even seeing if the patient does indeed want to heal themselves or even live for that matter. If a patient carries deep trauma, pain and guilt they may say they want to get better but their subconscious will betray all their "efforts" until the underlying cause of their dis-ease is rooted out and healed. Practitioners who have not gone down that dark inner path of facing their own inner shadows will not be able to assist others in this all important task. And if the co-healer fails to place the responsibility of wellness on the recipient's shoulders they ultimately will never experience true "holistic" healing.

We have reached a time on this planet where detoxing all the bodies is key to easing the flow of energy through the body and healing dis-ease. Our bodies are naturally being realigned to our divine natural state of wholeness or holiness. As we heal physically, emotionally, mentally and spiritually all our bodies will flow with ease as the divine energy of the Creator increases. Dis-ease will become a thing of the past. Health and well being will become our natural state of existence. Our bodies natural intuitive ways of regaining balance will become more and more the curative factor and we will learn to listen to our bodies to give it what it needs in each moment to heal and alchemize the daily energies. The treatments will become more subtle as we rise in vibration above the lower frequencies into the higher more subtle vibrations more aligned with The Creator. Our bodies will crave a life style more in harmony with the bio-rhythms of our Mother Earth. We will find our lives shifting. We may move to more pristine rural settings, eat more high vibrational foods even grow our own food. We will let our food and herbs be our medicine and use the sunlight to heal and realign ourselves. We can even learn to transmute the destructive manmade electro magnetic energies of 5G and become living examples of the motto if it doesn't kill you it makes you stronger!

Society teaches that the deterioration of the physical body, old age, disease and death are phases everyone must go through. Old age to many people means illness, weakness, senility, decay, pain, poverty, fear, loneliness, ugliness and despair. Why must that be so? Why couldn't you instead think of wellness, riches, beauty, mastership, patience and wisdom that can only come through the passage of linear time? These are the qualities society needs to emphasize in its senior citizens. The senior, reflective years of your life could be a time chosen to evolve yourself spiritually to new levels not possible as a young restless and evolving soul. By letting in more of the divine light and love energy that always surrounds you, new levels of consciousness become possible. As fully realized individuals who are following their soul's path, the senior years could be a time to share your wisdom and knowledge. Once you learn to step out of the social grid which, looks at the negative aspect of "becoming old," and encourages you to "act you age", you will realize the physical body is meant to last as long as you need it. Even the simple act of celebrating your own birthday is really a ritual to remind you that the clock is ticking and someday you must die.

So sooner or latter you will be facing death—the end of every thing! But the truth is there is no death! We are eternal beings. We were created to have a healthy dis-ease free body that serves us well as long as we had need it to carry out our unique soul mission. When our job is done we must face our own death without fear knowing the truth, it is simply a change of form. Our consciousness is simply being poured from one container that was best suited for your old life and job into another better adapted for your new job. Something like changing your Volkswagen bug for a four wheel drive jeep.. You wouldn't want to drag you VW bug up treacherous terrain when you go on a wilderness adventure would you? You were always meant to maintain full memory of all your identities or experiences as consciousness in different containers. These memories will return as your divine technology comes back on line. The problem is that the human has been conditioned to believe that the material world is all there is. This is going to poise a great problem as people who are afraid of old age and death will flock to the latest technology as an easy way to obtain youth and immortally. But at what price? Your soul?

Healthcare programs need to be redesigned to help its recipients maintain perfect health by stressing the value of preventive medicine and treatments that respect the physical body. Healthcare facilities also need to evolve into true healing centers. Historically, a hospital was seen as a place for healing, an institution whose sole function was to help individuals become whole again. How many of you think of hospitals as healing centers? Over the past twenty years the American culture has seen a tremendous change in the way hospitals provide medical services. Today, hospitals seem to have more in common with big business enterprises than healing centers. Profitability and work efficiency is where the focus lies. Large or small, the bottom line seems to be the same: profit. The public constantly hears the same propaganda: we provide excellent health care at reasonable costs. Although on the surface it sounds like a perfectly good motto, too often the emphasis shifts from patient care to profits. Who is defining good quality health care? What are their parameters? Is a hospital with a well trained staff of doctors, nurses, paramedical personnel, up to date technology and comfortable rooms considered an excellent medical institution?

According to most licensing authorities those three factors tell most of the story. But what about the patient? From the patient's perspective, is the facility composed of caring providers? Do they spend time explaining procedures, diagnoses and other general concerns the average patient may have? Do they empower patients by allowing them to assume an active role as co-healers in their own recovery? Or do they insist on making all the decisions? Is their primary goal to assist the individual in healing himself/herself, utilizing a variety of resources including medicines, technology, and nutritional counseling in a nurturing environment? Do you see the difference? During my training I (Peter), worked in hospitals considered by most people to be the best in the country. In retrospect, a key ingredient was lacking in these institutional Meccas: Love! Tender, loving care is not something you can buy, yet it is the most powerful healing force in existence. To doctors in training, patients were identified as dis- eases or cases, not as unique human beings facing a life crisis. What they needed most from us was love, respect and compassion. These were not emphasized as much as the pathophysiological course of the illness.

How many of you have ever been admitted to a hospital? I have. Although I have never been inside a prison, it felt like one. Employees coming in and out of my room constantly. Beepers and alarms going off at all hours, which kept me from getting what the doctor said I needed most: rest. The food was barely edible. The nursing personnel was always engaged in other activities, too busy to respond to my calls. The day I was finally discharged I thanked God I survived the experience! It is no wonder patients feel so depressed when they have to be admitted to the hospital. Most people know a hospital stay means not only having to contend with a serious illness, but also being treated in a humiliating fashion for the sake of expedience. This type of administration is diametrically opposed to the essence of a true healing center where expediency takes a back seat to helping the afflicted realign himself or herself to achieve wellness.

During a recent assignment in the Carolinas, I recall working in a small community hospital that was owned by a large corporation. Although I never had any contact with the administrator, all the employees displayed one very important component in the way they conducted their work: love. Everywhere in the hospital you could sense a caring attitude that was lacking in most famous medical centers. All the patients who stayed in this little hospital benefitted from this wonderful healing energy that filled the air. I remember working with a doctor who had not enjoyed a single day off in years, until I came to town to relieve him. I never heard him complain once about his workload and often wondered what drove him so feverishly to be of service to others. I knew money was not the motivator, since most of his patients were poor. He typified the general attitude of all caretakers associated with this hospital. Caring seemed to supersede all other ingredients such as medical technology or efficiency. The patients admitted to this hospital seemed to get well faster than the patients admitted to other larger, more technologically advanced institutions. The lesson I took home from this experience was that love and caring far exceeded any other form of treatment. This is precisely the reason I ponder the true meaning of such statements as, "We provide excellent healthcare at reasonable costs."

In the modern history of medicine, we have never before seen medical care being measured by a yardstick called money. This phenomenon is happening in every community. Human compassion seems to have taken a backseat to budgetary constraints. Who is to blame for this change in values? Are hospitals meant to function as businesses? Is good health a commodity only accessible to the rich? Managed Healthcare, which we will all be forced to contend with, inappropriately mixes cost efficiency and profitability with healthcare. These for-profit corporations were given permission by Congress to provide medical care to subscribers with the hope that the cost of services would be comparatively less than traditional medical insurance plans. Although most governmental authorities agree that Managed Healthcare has accomplished this goal, the trade off has been quality of care. These entities deliver facility based medical services by either having complete ownership of a hospital, or contracting with a local institution for a set number of beds at a fixed fee per category of dis- ease. The dilemma I often ran into as a provider was being forced to discharge a patient prematurely because the plan would not allow a longer stay in the hospital. Repeatedly, I felt the patient's best interest was not top priority in the decision making process.

More recently a new entity has risen in the healthcare arena. An agency enters a contract with a city to operate an entire hospital along with salaried medical, nursing and laboratory staff. The geographic location of this type of facility is usually found in an inner suburb or a remote town where trained personnel is difficult to obtain. This unchecked power to provide essential medical services, motivated solely by profit, has caused serious deficiencies in the quality of health care patients receive. Not long ago, I was forced to leave such a situation when I found out critically important surgical equipment had not arrived at the hospital I was serving. This hospital had recently been opened to serve a high risk suburb of a large Midwestern city. This abrupt decision to leave twenty-four hours after arrival created some personal financial difficulties, but I felt compelled to express my deepest concern to the managing director of the agency. His response was to seek the advice of other physicians employed there who unfortunately refused to reveal the seriousness of the situation for fear of financial repercussions. Privately they had agreed the risk of harming patients was high. The possibility of postponing the grand opening of the hospital until all necessary equipment had arrived was quickly dismissed as impractical and unnecessary.

As healthcare continues to evolve into a big business, individuals need to become more responsible about their own health. Many families have at some point in their lives dealt with the emotional and devastating financial consequences that a serious illness for one of the family members causes. One of the main factors leading to today's healthcare crisis is the cost of hospitalization. Even the cost of so called outpatient surgery where the patient remains in the hospital for not more than a few hours is astronomical.

In 1990 I had the opportunity to visit Germany for postgraduate surgical training and witnessed first hand how a social medical system operates. A noticeable difference was the scanty use of disposable items in the operating theater. By contrast, American hospitals seldom employ reusable instruments or other operating room paraphernalia. The social phenomenon of disposability has no better illustration than a typical operating suite in this country. Everything is disposable. Needless to say surgical instrument corporations and medical supply houses are flourishing, while society foots the enormous bill that hospitals send to the patients' insurance companies. A good example of the ridiculous state of affairs occurred when a former patient brought in her hospital bill that showed a ten dollar charge for a single Tylenol tablet.

Most hospitals receive payment for only a fraction of the total bill from both

Medicare and Medicaid. In most communities this accounts for the majority of patients. Private medical insurance companies and the uninsured patients end up pay ing for this humongous unnecessary waste. Reportedly, the reason for this heavy utilization of disposables is the prevention of communicable diseases and a lower operating room related infection rate. However, in Germany I worked in a three hundred year old medical institution where some of the most famous surgeons trained and there was no difference in the infection rate from re-sterilizing surgical instruments, gowns, sheets and so on.

One clinical example of this wastage is in performing a laparoscopic hysterectomy. In this country the procedure relies on the use of disposable clips that can add up to $4,000.00 to the hospital price tag. In Germany, a similar surgical procedure is performed for a total of a few hundred marks or several hundred dollars. Why waste so much money? Providing excellent health care does not mean employing the most expensive technology that often goes hand in hand with disposables. A hospital acting responsibly is one that respects the human body as a living temple and provides new technologies which are minimally invasive. It also uses good judgement in employing reusable equipment and supplies that respect the environment.

Hospitals were meant to be healing centers. Places where the patient is restored to perfect health by bringing more of the Creator's Light into the physical body through a process of purification or detoxification. This realignment is achieved by bringing into harmony all energy systems, bodily fluids and excretions utilizing a wide variety of techniques, therapies and practices. The individual needs to assume an active role in his/ her own healing. All members of the healing team are expendable except for the patient. Obviously their role is to empower the patient to self heal. This empowerment comes from shifting the ultimate responsibility of healing to the afflicted. The value of preventive medicine is emphasized by aiding individuals in the realization that for every action they take regarding the treatment of their bodies, there is an equal and opposite reaction. The healing team, led by the physician, will work with the patient through whatever unbalanced situation is going on in his/her daily lives that is manifesting in an illness. Unlike the present, where most physicians concern themselves with dis- ease processes and laboratory results, the primary interest will be placed on how the illness is affecting the individual as a whole. The plan of management will therefore be in taking corrective measures in lifestyle changes to prevent its recurrence. Other team members will carry on this focus of wholeness in their approach as health facilitators. Technology will be employed to the extent that it treats the physical body as a holy temple housing the spirit. Surgical intervention will emphasize respect for the physical vehicle and a greater degree of reliance on the body's natural healing powers. These modern technologies will be blended with ancient methods of healing to provide a new integrated and evolved practice of medicine. Understanding energy balancing, chakra systems and true ascension mechanics will also be incorporated into traditional medicine and mental health care to provide the best of both worlds and offer the patient a more extensive array of options.

As hospitals evolve their function, certain members of society will insist on following a path of self destruction refusing to accept any responsibility concerning their own health. Many will continue to abuse their bodies no matter what is taught to them. Many will opt to go for the "Quick Fix" of technology. Society must learn to exercise restrain and accept the reality that everyone has the inborn right of freewill and complete ownership of their own physical vehicle. It is not society's role to act as a parent when it comes to dealing with some of their own members. Likewise society no longer needs to make itself responsible for the health consequences of those bent on self destruction.

A good example to illustrate this point is the patient I cared for recently whom I delivered by cesarean. She developed toxemia of pregnancy, a unique illness usually associated with high blood pressure and neurological complications that can be devastating, even lethal. She had been diagnosed as hypertensive sometime before conceiving this pregnancy. The patient became quite ill during the labor process with an extremely elevated blood pressure and neurological manifestations of an impending life-threatening situation. Her social history revealed drug abuse confirmed by a urine screening test upon arrival to the hospital. The cesarean went well and a healthy boy, four weeks premature, was delivered. Over the following forty-eight hours her blood pressure rose which prompted a consultation with two internists to control the hypertensive crisis which we all feared could lead to a stroke or even death. On the morning of the third day the patient signed herself out of the hospital against medical advice. My colleagues and I were horrified by her actions which we suspected were drug related. A week later the patient showed up in the clinic with incredibly high blood pressure and was upset because the internists had refused to see her again. I sat her down and calmly reinforced the fact that she was the sole owner of her body and no one had the right to force her to do something against her will. She nodded in agreement. By the same token, choosing to leave the hospital prematurely as she did, signified to all of us that she was assuming total responsibility for her own health. Acting against medical advice removed all responsibility from our shoulders. As it stands to date under modern American medico-legal rules, this patient becomes the responsibility of the hospital if she is brought in by ambulance suffering from a stroke as a consequence of her irresponsible behavior. Is society acting responsibly by forcing hospitals to provide medical care to individuals who act in such a manner?

By comparison, another patient comes to mind who is twenty three years old and suffers excruciating pain with every menstrual cycle. I was highly suspicious of endometriosis. This is a dis- ease that causes inflammation of the pelvis and infertility. I recommended a laparoscopy to inspect the pelvis and begin treatment as soon as possible. Unfortunately, she had no insurance and although the clinic where I was temporarily employed would allow me to perform the surgery at no charge, the local hospital refused to provide care because of lack of funds. As far as the system is concerned, this patient's condition is not life threatening so therefore, under the law, the hospital can deny services. When I compare the two patients and consider the limited financial resources available to the needy, I immediately see the system's inadequacies.

Healthcare could shift to create healing centers that will have open and outdoor structures that reflect a balanced relationship of nature and architecture optimizing the healing energy. Hospitals could be situated in a nature oriented setting and constructed in a way to maximize light and greenery and the bio rhythms of the grounds harmoniously aligning patients to drink in its healing effects by allowing more Light frequencies to come in contact with patients. The natural healing process could thus be maximized. Nutrition, herbal supplements and balancing treatments would play a key role in the center. These healing centers could become teaching learning retreats where indigenous leaders could share their ancient knowledge and help humankind find their way back home. As co-healers and patients work together, wellness will be restored by promoting the body's own natural healing powers. Patients will be counseled in all four aspects of their being: physical, mental, emotional and spiritual natures, as preventive medicine becomes the main focus of the new healthcare system in our world.

EHS (electromagnetic hypersensitivity) has at long last found its way into modern medicine as a recognized dis-ease. However these EMF sensitive folks (Elizabeth) myself included, are the Canaries in the Coal Mind warning us of what is coming. Healthcare practitioners looking for temporally solutions so people can continue their dis-eased life styles in our modern man made world of increasing EMF toxicity are throwing "shield and heal" solutions at the public. People are scrambling to protect their homes and families from the devastating effects of 5G radiation coming not only from cell towers but now emitted from satellites in the Space X cage. As the EMF protection and health supplementation industries' profits sore, Smart Cities are being created encapsulating human beings with electrical A.I. networks. If this unchecked expansion is not stopped the only way people will be able to survive in these modern AI environments is to become AI life forms themselves! Many will allow themselves to be deceived thinking AI has been made SAFE and is the cure for all humankind's problems rather than see it a symptom of a world living outside of the Will of the Divine Creators and ITS Natural Laws. They will choose the easy path that will not require them to take responsibility for their own physical, emotional, mental and spiritual health and well being. They will see technology as the cure to all the woes of the world and be herded into a false Artificial ascension matrix.

It is becoming apparent that 5G and this rapid technological expansion is the cancer, a dis-ease of modern man. Perhaps to regain balance we need to take a few steps backwards and heed the wisdom of the ancients we have cast aside in our rush towards "progress" and return to living in harmony with the organic electromagnetic bio rhythms of nature. Perhaps our indigenous brothers and sisters can remind us how to live in harmony with the our Mother Earth and our own inner divine technology will come back on line. But this is something the modern "white" man does not want to do. They have not been heeding the signs that our dis-eased Mother Earth and our native brothers and sister have been giving to us. Instead we have killed off our indigenous brothers and sisters replacing their wisdom with the latest propaganda piece on media (both mainstream and alternative).

It will be those who can realign themselves and assist others to realign themselves with the natural bio rhythms of our ascending Sun, Mother Earth and "easily" flow with the Divine Will of the our Infinite Creator who will "cure" the Dis- Ease of our World. Those who understand the TRUTH of our current global heath crisis and that C.O.V.I.D is simply a symptom of the greater dis- ease of Humankind's separation from their Divine Creator. They will be the ones who will be the new Co-healor who will help others do what they themselves have done. As this happens humanity can reposition itself away from its dis-eased state and back into the ease of flowing in alignment with the Creator and our Mother Earth. The indigenous people of our Earth have stored this ancient knowledge for eons. We modern dis-eased humans have much to learn from their "store"-ries". But will we listen?

A.I. "Artificial" Intelligence is the symptom of the dis-eased state of our world. Our world that has completely forgotten what is real. We have replaced Artificial Intelligence with Divine Intelligence. We have made technology our God the Artificial Creator rather than the Divine Intelligence of the Infinite Creator. We are spending more and more of our time and energy living in an Artificial world not even noticing how our own world is becoming faker by the moment, filled with fake food (GMO) fake clothing, fake relationships. We are spending more and more of our precious time "online" in a cyber world inside a "Net" where we no longer, touch, taste, smell, or feel. Where everything is fake. We are not seeing that our forests are gone, our rivers and oceans are poisoned, our land is barren and our birds and bees are dying! Many of us seldom go outdoors and feel the wind on our face, the earth beneath our feet, pick an apple from a tree, embrace another human being. Many of us do not spend time with their own children letting the AI world raise them. What are we becoming? What are our children becoming? Many who are not finding a balance between the man made Artificial world of AI and the real organic world the Creator created are beginning to experience dis-ease as a warning sign. The Cure for this A.I. dis-ease is to return to living in harmony with our Mother Earth, nature and the Will of the Divine Creators. Artificial technology (AI) is a stepping stone to your own inner Divine Inner Technology! Use it wisely to serve you, not you to serve it! Use it for your soul mission and dis-ease as a warning sign to ground yourself in the Real World of Organic Life.

THE HOPI PROPHECY

Thomas Banyacya explains in two timely talks from 1995, how: three previous human worlds were destroyed when people became greedy, worshiped technology as their God, fought and hurt each other, and repeatedly forgot the ethical teachings they'd been given to honor the Earth as the source of life and sustenance. Elder Grandfather Martin Gashweseoma, who interprets the Prophecy Rock, speaks of two paths, the top path is of the two hearted people that everyone thinks is the right path and follows, then there is the second path of truth that leads to everlasting life that only a few one hearted people follow. The top line ends abruptly while the bottom line continues around the rock.

THE WARRIORS OF THE RAINBOW: HOPI PROPHECY

"One day... there would come a time, when the earth being ravaged and polluted, the forests being destroyed, the birds would fall from the air, the waters would be blackened, the fish being poisoned in the streams, and the trees would no longer be, mankind as we would know it would all but cease to exist...a new tribe of people shall come unto the earth from many colors, classes, creeds and who by their actions and deeds shall make the earth green again. This tribe shall be called The Warriors of the Rainbow and it will put its faith in actions not words. They will move over the Earth like a great Whirling Rainbow, bringing peace, understanding and healing everywhere they go. We will learn how to see and hear in a sacred manner. Men and women will be equals in the way Creator intended them to be; all children will be safe anywhere they want to go. Elders will be respected and valued for their contributions to life. Their wisdom will be sought out. The whole Human race will be called "The People" and there will be no more war, sickness or hunger forever. If the New People remain strong in their quest, the sacred drum will again sound its voice. There will be an awakening of the people, and the sacred fire will again be lit. At this time, the light-skinned race will be given a choice between two roads. One road is the road of greed and technology without wisdom or respect for life. This road represents a rush to destruction. The other road is spirituality, a slower path that includes respect for all living things. If we choose the spiritual path, we can light yet another fire, an Eighth Fire, and begin an extended period of Peace and healthy growth."

What most people fail to understand is that our Mother Earth is on an autocorrection course of restoring balance and curing this A.I. Dis-Ease of modern man. It is the responsibility of each individual to decide if they want to heal themselves by restoring balance and moving with ease onto a higher timeline in harmony with the Divine Intelligence of organic life, nature and our Mother Earth or do they want to continue on their destructive path worshipping Artificial technology A.I. as their God? The choice is yours... choose wisely.

Section Four:

Social And Financial Evolvment

Societal institutions that thrive on the use of power and greed will crumble as the planet moves into the 5th dimension.

CHAPTER 8
GREED (IN AMERICA)

As your physical, emotional, mental and spiritual natures evolve and equilibrate, you are ready to begin evolving socially and financially. Your emotional body will then give way to financial and social evolvement. Think of yourself as a being with spirituality represented as the head, mental and physical natures as the arms and financial and social natures as the legs. Your job is to evolve all natures equally. The problem in the Western hemisphere is that too much emphasis is placed on evolving financially without first bringing the other four natures into balance. Everything begins with spirituality. If you have your spirituality in place, all the other natures will evolve, including financial and social in a harmonious way.

Everything begins with spirituality. If you have your spirituality in place, all the other natures will evolve, including financial and social in a harmonious way.

Have you ever seen someone who is extremely wealthy, but miserable? Perhaps they are paranoid about people cheating them out of their money, or maybe their personal life is in shambles. If your wealth does not bring you peace of mind, what good is it? Is this true financial abundance? Financial abundance is the frosting on the cake, the jewel in your crown, which arrives with ease when all other natures are in order. It comes from the joy of self expression, self discovery and being of service. How many people have you known who have come by a sum of money in a dishonest way and kept that money? The law of Karma will always prevail although it may take linear time, eventually, these people always pay back. The money will either be lost in poor investments, stolen, or just spent unwisely. Money earned through service and invested with wisdom will grow and bring fruits of abundance to its investor. Money, like an abundance of food, should be shared wisely when you are fulfilled.

Unfortunately, it seems greed is the principal thought form in the marketplace today. Greed is a dis- ease that plagues those who live by it with the never ending pain of never having enough. Greedy people can never experience the joy of abundance because they can never have enough wealth, enough material possessions, enough food, enough sex, etc. There is always a great emptiness within them that cannot be filled since it comes from feeling disconnected from the Creator. Endlessly, these folks look to the material world for fulfillment. Until they realize they cannot buy the things they want most: peace of mind, love, health, youth, etc. They may die having the most toys but what have they really won? The material world is an illusion that people often become lost in. The best way to illustrate how greed blocks spiritual unfoldment for the individual/group/country/planet is to look at the institutions within a country that clearly function at that level and examine how this incorrect thinking affects its citizens.

Since I (Peter), am a physician, it is easiest for me to start with my own profession. It is unfortunate to see how far from true healing most physicians' offices are in today's society. It is not hard to recognize that most medical practices focus on the business aspect rather than the healing aspect of the job. Many physicians are doing a great job in this arena to the detriment of most patients. Third party payers and even government insurance programs are set up in such a way as to force physicians to deal with quantity of care rather than quality of care. In the struggle to make a lucrative living, patients are treated in the most efficient way to treat a specific physical complaint and are discharged from care as quickly as possible. The idea of holistic medicine is totally lost in the expediency to match some illness to a proper code which insurance companies use as the bible to reimburse physicians (and hospitals as well). What about the patient? Is treating a specific symptom going to achieve a lasting wellness in that patient?

An incident comes to mind illustrating this point which involved a patient referred to me by a busy internist in a small community. The patient was a young woman who apparently developed a large tumor in one of her ovaries. After examining the patient and discussing different treatment options with her, she and I decided surgery was necessary to remove the tumor. I then called the referring physician to assist in the surgery but it seemed no time was convenient for him. He offered several excuses that included conflicts with either the office schedule or his day off. I finally decided to do the surgery myself with the assistance of other nursing personnel. A few weeks later the same physician referred another patient to me with exactly the same problem except she was older than the previous patient. This time I did not bother calling him when the patient was scheduled for surgery, although I did ask for his consultation regarding the management of her diabetes and hypertension. Afterwards, the physician angrily approached me and asked why I had not invited him to assist in the surgery of "his patient." Later the reason for the inconsistent behavior became apparent: The first patient had no medical insurance. The second one did. This man illustrates where many physicians are today and how far from the original concept of healing the medical profession has come. It is obvious from this man's behavior that his judgement has been consumed by greed as his medical practice is simply the means by which he can make lots of money.

Another area within the field of healthcare which is an example of greed biasing the decisions participants make is medical malpractice. Even medical experts cannot agree on how much money medical malpractice is costing the nation today. Part of the problem is trying to come up with a reliable figure concerning the way physicians are forced to practice their craft to avoid a potential lawsuit. This is what is known as practicing defensive medicine.

It is virtually impossible to calculate how many unnecessary tests and other precautionary measures physicians take on a daily basis since many of these additional steps have been integrated into the practice of modern medicine. After a while these tests become part of the "standard practice of medicine" and it then becomes risky for a physician to deviate from the "norm," and so the test is added to the roster of others. Two examples to illustrate this point are intrapartum fetal heart rate monitoring for a normal patient in labor and screening mammography for women under fifty years of age. In both cases the test has not been shown to benefit patients and yet millions of dollars continue to be spent on a daily basis largely because hospitals and physicians are afraid of being sued.

A question to ask at this point is, if patients are not benefiting from these expensive measures, then who is? The answer is obvious: attorneys. Just as the physician I described earlier who cared more about making money than the welfare of his patients, some malpractice attorneys are making millions of dollars a year from the suffering of patients. This does not mean that a physician or any person should not be held accountable for negligent actions, but greed has caused lawyers to abuse the system.

Can anyone know for certain why things happen the way they do sometimes? How would you judge an earthquake occurring and killing 10,000 people? How about a tidal wave drowning another 10, 000 human beings? Most people would say those events are different because as natural disasters no one can be blamed. These events are not judged according to societal rules, and yet, these incidents still go on happening and devastating members of our species. Why should we employ a separate set of rules to judge an unfavorable event that causes misery or even death to someone, if no malice or negligence is intended? How are these events different from each other? There are no accidents. Everything happens for a reason, so in the end, who can really say why somebody got hurt?

A national system of compensation needs to be established to pay for whatever hospitalization costs or other related healthcare services are needed to care for the injured party. Regrettably, a nofault healthcare compensation system such as the one I described does not exist today. Instead the medicolegal climate functions like a lottery. The emphasis is being placed on monetary compensation which largely benefits the attorneys in lieu of support systems to help the injured party. Apparently greed rules most of the decisions being made in this arena and thus malpractice lawsuits have become one of the main contributing factors in the healthcare crisis facing the country today.

The area of banking similarly illustrates how greed takes center stage. A good example is how the Federal Reserve System came into being. It is interesting to see how a small group of powerful men were able to convince Congress as far back as 1791 that a Central Bank was needed to control the money supply and thus, in their opinion, stabilize the nation's economy. The interesting part of this story is that these men controlled 80% of the stocks that were initially issued with the federal government only owning 20% of the total shares. In other words, a small group of private citizens (bankers) were in control of the money supply for the entire population. Over the next forty years enough members of Congress kept this elite group from interfering with the affairs of the nation. In 1832, president Andrew Jackson vetoed a bill that would have renewed the Central Bank and instead spear headed a policy of hard currency which meant every paper note was backed by either silver or gold. By January 1835 president Jackson had paid off the national debt thus becoming the only president ever to do so.

But the story does not end there. This powerful band of elite men continued their unrelenting effort and in 1913, backed by other faceless international and equally powerful individuals, they won a major victory and a Central Bank disguised under a new name was born. This is how the Federal Reserve Act came into being. It is crucially important for anyone who cares about the welfare of this country to understand the immense significance of this "federal" body. A small group of bankers, direct descendants of the most powerful families in this country, with the help of other European friends, also descendants of equally powerful families in their countries, were given the license to print as much money as they felt the country needed. To give you an example of where these people were coming from, by the year 1989 the national debt was three trillion dollars. More than half of what all Americans paid in their federal income tax returns went straight into the pockets of these bankers to pay for the interest on this multitrilliondollar loan. Who are these men? How can it be that a few unelected private citizens can have so much power?

Most political historians will agree that the first step toward controlling a country is to issue credit to its citizens. The more you owe them, the more they own you. If this statement is true, then most of you are owned by a small group of bankers who choose to remain anonymous except to a few individuals in key government positions who follow their orders. What can you expect from an institution whose leaders are solely motivated by greed? Remember in the 1980's how many banks went under and why? Greed. What about today? Do you see a change of policy in the way most banks operate?

An interesting event took place a few months ago when I (Peter), went to the bank and noticed a sign that stated they were moving soon. I asked the teller why they were moving. She replied, "We're consolidating with another branch two miles away." I was puzzled by her answer since this particular branch always seemed busy and it would certainly be an inconvenience to many customers to travel an extra two miles to do their banking. With some sadness in her face she replied

"Well, they really want to replace most of us (tellers) with ATM machines." Her answer made it all too clear, banks are replacing people that need to be paid salaries and benefits with machines that stay open 24 hours a day and often charge customers for the convenience of withdrawing their own money. In other words, they save salaries and make more money with their machines. Do you get the picture?

In fact, the worst part is that most other institutions work the same way: money first, service last. Insurance companies are a prime example of this. It started out as a good idea which was for people to pool their money together so that in the event a member of the group experienced a disaster, s/he would have the financial resources to recover. The problem occurred when these companies grew larger and became more impersonal. At this point, answering the profit demands of investors, they began to invest their monetary reserves in order to pay dividends. As the years went by, they amassed huge amounts of wealth and lost sight of their original purpose by letting greed rule their decision to settle claims. Have you ever tried to collect on an insurance claim? Many people have to hire attorneys to force these huge corporations to live up to their agreement. Certainly there is insurance fraud in America, but which came first?

Many corporations, professional athletes, entertainment icons, religious institutions, hospitals and communication services are other examples of where the sense of service and responsibility toward others has been replaced with greed. The quest for money (paper unbacked by silver or gold) is the main driving force behind most business decisions made today. Meanwhile these bankers who remain faceless, privately become richer and more powerful while most people are being squeezed by the shrinking real money supply (backed by silver and gold). Their agenda is right on schedule, is yours?

The time has come for you to wake up from the dream and realize what is going on around you. You must start now to take charge of your life by making a conscious decision not to be a pawn. One organization we belonged to in Arizona was a food coop. It was a member owned organization whose goal was to provide the highest quality of food for the lowest price. This is in direct contrast to how most businesses operate. Cooperatives could serve as models for other services rendered to members such as banking, insurance needs, community farming, etc. The point is, we need to come together in cooperation, not competition.

The first step in getting off the train is always the hardest but then it becomes easier. Reduce your spending and get back to basics. Early in my spiritual journey I (Peter), once asked my teacher: "Why is it I can't seem to get out of debt?" He replied, "You're telling me you still have many desires." Pay off your debts and learn to live in simplicity. Use credit cards as little as possible and pay them off quickly. Do not let greed continue to rule your life.

During these times societal systems are sinking under their own bureaucratic weight and failing to provide for those who need help. As baby boomers grow closer to retirement, the financial strain on Social Security and Medicare assistance programs are rapidly reaching bankruptcy levels. This social dilemma is coming to the awareness of future recipients who feel the government has failed them and consequently find themselves victims to a social system they helped create and have supported financially. Current retirees are already feeling the crunch of the shrinking dollar. My (Peter), own mother illustrates this by needing financial assistance from family members and having to work a part time job at eighty years of age to meet monthly expenses. The feeling of uncertainty often fills her mind as she tries to make ends meet. On a larger scale the country is trying to find its place as a global recession looms over the heads of many working citizens already barely able to keep up with expenses and unable to save for their own retirement or to subsidize future social security payments. Most Americans are in debt and sinking deeper into financial instability. The chaotic state of affairs creates great concern for the many individuals, like my mother, who banked on social systems to help them and instead feel the burden of the bureaucracy financed by their own tax dollars.

Recently I watched a classic movie made by Frank Capra entitled "You Can't Take It With You." It's a good flick to rent out and see what I'm talking about. Life's most beautiful things are free. The simpler, more detached from the physical world you are, the closer you will be to God. To best evolve financially one must learn to depend on the sense of intuition and practice self reliance adhering to the principle of keep it simple. As you learn to focus internally a greater sense of awareness will reach your consciousness and external events will seem unimportant when compared to your own inner peacefulness. This is not to say you loose interest in life and what goes on around you. On the contrary, as you practice equanimity and detachment from the physical world, a constant sense of well being replaces old beliefs that promote dependency on external objects and systems. No longer will you have to buy your dream house or drive a particular car, or vacation in a particular place. The "keep up with the Jones" lifestyle will give way to financial liberation. This does not mean you renounce your worldly possessions, but it could help to lighten up! Get rid of the junk. When you buy something that you really need and will use, buy the best. When you work, do your job out of a sense of service, not constantly looking for rewards financially or otherwise. This does not mean you don't get a pay check, obviously you need to make money, but rather than placing your emphasis on financial gain, look at what you are learning from the experience, no matter how mundane the task may seem. As you do this you will come from a place of joy, knowing that you are fulfilling your purpose.

The old saying that proclaims there is beauty in simplicity is best suited for the area of financial evolvement, as opposed to the complicated situations that often draw the individual deeper into debt and the emotional turmoil associated with it. Let go of the illusion of making a million dollars and retiring to a tropical island. Place your emphasis on service and self discovery rather than on monetary gain and financial abundance will be yours unlike those who have made money their God. Life becomes a journey full of surprises and tests designed to help you evolve physically, mentally, emotionally, spiritually. . . and financially and socially. As you evolve in all natures it will become apparent that societal institutions such as government are not conforming to the principles that created them. It is our duty as concerned citizens to examine this powerful institution carefully and do our best to bring our expanded awareness into it.

CHAPTER 9

GOVERNMENT AND POWER

In searching for the seed to write this chapter, the image of a dollar bill kept flashing into my mind. I (Peter), finally took one and studied it carefully. To me, the most impressive part of the dollar was the phrase written on the back which reads "In God we trust." I noticed that the same words were written on every paper note no matter what the denomination was. Those are very powerful and symbolic words: The people of this nation trust in God. We the people, you and me and the other two hundred and sixty million U.S. Citizens who live across this land, have trusted the government to preserve our individual rights; we have believed our government officials have been making decisions in our best interest and that they are serving, and following the Divine Will of God.

The republic of the United States of America is defined as a state in which the supreme power rests in the body of citizens entitled to vote and is exercised by representatives and states men, chosen directly or indirectly by the body of citizens. When you think of the government, what comes into your mind? Authority? Power? Fear? Control? Politics? Taxes? Military? Weapons? Bureaucracy? Waste? Do you perhaps think of representatives serving a body of citizens? The Constitution states that we are all created equal, which signifies that our founding fathers were inspired by a higher principle. Collectively they made a resolution to create a place on this planet where all men and women could evolve physically, emotionally, mentally and spiritually without interference from government. This foundation is based on the sovereignty of its people. No matter what race, creed, skin color, or religion, inherent in our Constitution is the right of self-expression: the right to be the authority of your life, and free-dome, the dome being the dome of your head, thus enabling you to have a free head to think independently and to speak your mind freely. Is this the way our government is working today? Do you sometimes get the feeling of being a grain of sand in a huge desert in the middle of a storm, or perhaps you feel like cattle being herded and prodded to the tune of someone else's whim?

The highest spiritual focus a government can have is to promote self-governing practices and to encourage individuals to be responsible for themselves. But we the people must merit this freedom by acting responsibly. When the people of a nation refuse to act responsibly or to take the time to supervise the people whom they have elected to govern, they leave themselves wide open for a corrupt government to take their freedom away, until one day the precious freedom they took for granted is no longer there.

Since its conception this country has opted for the use of force as the predominant means to expand its physical borders. With war after war the government became more powerful, more selfserving and less attentive to its primary function: to serve its citizens. The end result is "we the people" have allowed this incredibly powerful institution to grow into its enormous size and now we find ourselves servants to it rather than it to us.

Some would say the way a democracy works is by majority rule. If a particular individual finds him/herself in the minority, well then that's too bad—majority rules. To be self-governing, however, symbolizes the individual citizen having the innate right, under God, to follow his/her pursuit of happiness without interference from others. This rule always applies unless the individual, while exercising this right, forces his/her will upon others. Even if only a single citizen takes a stand on a particular issue, under the Constitution that citizen cannot be denied his/her right to a voice. The conflict we commonly see is when a citizen, while exercising his/her human rights, takes a position that opposes a prevailing law. As the government becomes more complex, those simple words written in the Constitution which allow everyone the freedom to pursue happiness, are lost in the maze of laws added to the books year after year. It is obvious these new laws generally give the government more selfautonomy, creating a new layer of bureaucrats to enforce them, requiring more taxes. The Constitution was designed by our forefathers to insure that our rights would prevail even if our government should fall into the hands of a few corrupt individuals. This very Constitution is in danger of being lost.

Do you feel powerless when it comes to dealing with the government? Did you ever try to convince some governmental office about something that was adversely affecting you or a loved one? It is an impossible task, is it not? A bureaucrat will cite several rules that forbid you from doing something you feel very strongly about. These individuals are also part of "We the people." The problem is that they have forgotten how to move from a place of compassion and responsibility instead of worrying about their own individual needs such as job security or pensions. Because of the illusion of separateness, a division is occurring between those who support and/or are employed by the government and those who feel threatened by it. (Please notice we have stopped referring to it as our government).

A government cannot possibly control a nation unless the people of that nation carry out their orders. Most citizens in this country have been raised to not ask questions and to do what they are told, often following orders coming from a place of fear where the government is concerned. Military training is based on this very principal and drilled into the minds of all who participate in it. Even outside the military the same mentality prevails where corporate employees follow orders and refuse to think. When you question a ruling, the only way to make a point is to ask for a supervisor, or someone who can think. Love and compassion for others supersedes anybody's rules. It is your responsibility to know what is really going on around you. Refusing to find out or to see the truth of things does not insulate you from being held accountable by a higher order.

This does not mean you should avoid government positions or work in the military. We need people who can make a difference. We need individuals who can hold positions of power but do not get lost in them. If everyone who is virtuous and spiritually oriented remains outside the system how is government ever going to change? The only way this powerful institution can evolve is to dissolve the illusion of separateness. By changing from within and remaining focused on reaching Godrealization, you will emanate all the blessings that go with that goal such as virtue, compassion, expanded awareness and above all, the ability to set a living example to others.

In ancient Greek and in Shakespearean tragedies the powerful leader, usually a King, succumbs to defeat because of a flaw within his character. We must seek out our character flaws and fortify them. If we are not performing our duties as parents and instead expect the government to raise and educate our children, then future generations will pay the consequences. If we are so spiritually disconnected that we look to drugs or alcohol for our comfort, then the government will justify their right to set up road blocks and search our car. By using violence to solve family conflicts, the government will remove the right to bear arms and set up curfews with military supervision. With each act of irresponsibility we give more of our freedom to the government, who is all too willing to take it. You must dispense with the fairy tale that Uncle Sam is taking care of his little children. Know what you are looking at!

At present it would appear as if "the powers that be" have won. Corruption, greed cruelty, and suppression reign supreme. Many citizens feel powerless in the face of the government. If you succumb to these thoughts then they have you just where they want you. Remember you cannot control a person's soul. The government only has as much power over you allow them to have. "Give to Caesar what is Caesar's, and to God what is God's." In other words, let the government play its petty power games and don't lose sight of who you are and where you are going. Those who seek the truth and long for a world filled with peace, harmony and love must go within to find their inner truth.

In Italy the Italians have developed a strong sense of skepticism towards any government. People's loyalty is to their families and neighbors before their government which they know to be corrupt and not harboring their best interests. I am reminded of a delightful World War II movie, set in a small town in Italy where I (Elizabeth), spent much time. People in Italy are very intuitive. In this movie the Germans tried to steal wine from a small village famous for its unique vintage. The entire town pulled together and hides the wine in a cave, all the while appearing very helpful and compliant with the Germans.

The entire town pulled together and hid the wine in a cave, all the while appearing very helpful and compliant with the Germans. The German command was quite distressed by the fact they could not control these creative, innovative, and unified people. This is precisely the key to freedom.

Another example is the work of the great soul Mahatma Gandhi whose spiritual guidance and creative solutions lead an entire nation out of the bonds of British domination. Peaceful and unified resistance, not bloodshed, accomplished this goal. It is not a new event in history to see power hungry individuals abusing the governmental system to dominate the people of a nation. This weary human drama has been playing itself out for millenniums. What is new is the concept of escaping the Wheel of Karma by not being drawn in, feeling powerless and answering one act of violence with another.

As a boy growing up in Cuba, a country plagued by one bloody revolt after another, I (Peter), witnessed first hand the effects of political violence. First, I remember Castro over throwing Batista and watching the bloody executions Castro carried out, and then the many uprisings against him. I recall hearing of boyhood friends who had been taken in the night by the government and never heard from again.

Violence begets violence. Freedom born from violence has many karmic repercussions as we Americans are now finding out. It is easy for our incredibly technologically advanced government to wipe out any band of resistance. Movies like "Patriot Games" and "Undersiege II" expose the government's highly advanced satellites which can do anything from spying on nude sunbathers to creating devastating earthquakes. The only weapon powerful enough to stop the government is public opinion. This is the true power of the people. It's no wonder the government is trying to censor the film and television industry. Wars are won by the media and popularity polls. It is most difficult to control people who are creative and free thinkers. When you fight against a dominating force, it is easy for that force to over power you. The Aikido Master knows how to use the force of his/her aggressor to his/her benefit. By being creative, imaginative, and independent in thoughts and actions, you become much harder to control. That is why creativity and imagination are the first things to be removed from a society which is being controlled. If you allow yourself to be polarized by conflict you have given away your inner peace.

Government officials must realize their primary function is to serve the people. This message needs to be clearly sent to all our statesmen in Washington, D.C. The sacred oath taken by every member of government must be honored in the performance of all activities and duties. Much like the oath I (Peter), took when becoming a physician—to help others in times of need and to do no harm. They too need to remember, above all else, that their primary function is to serve the people and represent their individual rights—not only special interest groups that pay well. It is no wonder being a politician has become synonymous with such terms as corruption, deceit and greed. The once highly respected profession of statesman has descended to what it is now, an opportunity to abuse the trust of others for personal gain and power. Everyone jokes about the dishonesty of politicians, but it really is no laughing matter. We are distracted and divided by the dualistic illusion of democrats and republicans. If the truth be told there is little difference between the two parties since both have stopped serving the people. People talk about the upcoming presidential elections as choosing between the lesser of two evils. How did our current political system deteriorate to this point?

Imagine for one moment if all the citizens of the United States decided, at the same time, to stop supporting the federal government by ceasing to pay taxes. Despite the consequences, when the Internal Revenue Service sent their notices everyone unanimously said "No!" My guess is, within a short period of time, perhaps a few weeks, the government would collapse. Can you then imagine what the world would be like? Can you now appreciate how the government touches every aspect of your life? Over the years you have come to depend on the federal government for so much, it is unimaginable to think, even for a moment, how our society would survive with out their intervention. The point I am trying to illustrate is that all of us have allowed the government to become so expansive it presently controls every aspect of our society.

Another way to illustrate your dependency on the government is to imagine that a large meteor hits our country and millions of people were devastated by the consequences of such a tragic event. Are you living a life independent of government support? How many of you have your own well? How many of you grow your own food supply? How many of you are prepared to face such a disaster? It is only when you imagine these extreme life circumstances that you immediately realize your dependency on services now provided by various governmental agencies. Some of you may feel it is comforting to know the government is always there ready to provide at a moment's notice; constantly on guard, making all the decisions for us.

The fact is you are responsible adults meant to take care of your own affairs. The institution of government was created because individuals did not want the responsibility of making their own decisions. Regrettably in institutions like government, power is no longer where it belongs: in the hands of the individual citizen. Even now the government is trying to pass a law that will give it the authority to act as parents and decide what children can or cannot watch on television. This is the excuse they give for wanting to install chips into television sets that will sensor certain programs. Can you imagine other more sinister applications to these chips?

Even if their intentions were completely honorable and they were only wanting to shield children from violence, is it the government's job to supervise our children? Whatever happened to parents being the parent? When you take away a person's job, in this case the job of parenting, you take away that person's freedom. At first it may seem like they are doing you a favor, but the fact is you need the freedom to learn about yourself even if it means through mistakes. Individually and collectively you can change your government to function as it was meant to function: to serve the interests of its people.

One of the many responsibilities passed on to the government is national security. Under this label, individual rights guaranteed under the Constitution have suffered countless violations over the past three decades. To maintain national security, the government employs millions of citizens at a tremendous cost to the rest of the nation. This institution has also developed huge arsenals of deadly weapons capable of destroying the planet many times over. Does the government need all this force? Why must the government persist in believing it is responsible for the rest of the world? Does it have the right to interfere with another nation's sovereignty? Does the principle of a New World Order give it permission to dictate what other people do with their lives?

According to this concept, national borders are no longer respected by the United Nations security council and troops are dispatched to any part of the globe where in the opinion of those members, "order needs to be restored." The veil of secrecy seems to extend over many governmental activities presumably with the intent of protecting citizens from some foreign source. Civilian surveillance is commonplace, often with the individual unaware that his/her privacy is being invaded. Who really knows what goes on behind all this cloak and dagger? Does your intuition tell you something is amiss when it comes to the way government presently conducts its affairs? If for any reason a state of Marshall law is declared, this government would have complete and total control and all personal freedom would be suspended. If we proceed in the current direction the government is taking us, all military and other governmental agencies will possess the most technologically advanced firepower and the citizens of this nation will be armed with pepper gas.

The Vietnam War was a clear example how blind patriotism turned sour. Naively trusting the government and following orders to please king and country can have devastating effects. To the disappointment of many of those who made it back home, often showing mental, physical, emotional, and spiritual wounds from battle, they learned they had been pawns of politicians ruling the battlefields. Many of these vets felt empty and stressed to the point of not being able to function as productive citizens because of the atrocities they witnessed. Instead of finding the aid and comfort they sought in their homeland, they were regarded as politically incorrect and their emotional problems and war experiences largely ignored.

To be branded a coward or unpatriotic is a sensitive area that many male Americans have painfully learned are labels that carry with them tremendous negative social stigma. Nowadays, it is easy to be labeled as a coward if you choose not to give up God's most precious gift (your physical body) in raising arms against another group of individuals who disagree with the government's political views. War is glorified at some level by many members of society who feel the honor that is bestowed upon the individual defending his country is worth the price of his life.

The truth is all wars are political, so the question to ask is: Are you willing to kill another member of your species or lose your present carnation fighting for a political cause? If the answer is yes, because of your own reasons or personal agenda, then by all means do so. On the other hand, if you are uncertain about your own feelings, then you better think twice as karmically someone else's agenda will become your own if you decide to become part of a conflict. Often society (the government) does not allow the individual to make a personal choice (draft) and consequently many find them selves part of a conflict they were not supposed to be in. Many veterans of past wars learned this painful lesson and became incapacitated in some way trying to meet someone else's goal only to discover that in the end all that matters is what you think about yourself. This is not to say that sometimes, as was the case with Hitler, nations need to rally together in a common cause. Certainly, here one can argue the perceived reality (a single individual who wanted to rule the world) clearly left no room for anyone else who disagreed with his beliefs. Historically however, the agenda of a few individuals seeking personal power, all too often becomes (according to societal rules) the agenda of the followers. By abusing their positions, whether they happen to be kings, popes, wealthy bankers, prime ministers, presidents and so on, the result is that countless individuals either loose their most precious gift or become emotionally or physically incapacitated when societal rules (the draft) make it extremely difficult to choose not to fight.

The lesson to take home from the subject of patriotism is that the original intent of government is to promote self government. As you decide for yourself to become a participant in a national or global conflict, keep this principle in mind and see if it fits with your own agenda. Too often misguided individuals who mean well get caught in situations they later come to regret causing tremendous internal conflict which can manifest in serious and debilitating dis- eases.

Historically our nation has evolved aggressively, greedily gobbling up land that belonged to the indigenous tribes that were here before us and used dishonesty in breaking peace treaties signed with the Native Americans. Stealing Africans from their native lands to serve as slaves, and exploiting immigrant workers who arrived here seeking a better life was common place. Domination, injustice, and cruelty have been the birthing pains of this nation's history. This does not mean we lack the capacity to use our softness and forge a new course into the future. We must heal the gaping wounds of racism, injustice, and inequality and harmonize ourselves as a unit. We must learn to stop separating each other according to race, social class, religion, and geographical region and become a true melting pot extracting the highest essence from each culture. Even as Americans we must think more broadly and see ourselves as world citizens. We must see the highest essence of the New World Order, not as a few powerful men (bankers) trying to control all the wealth and power of the world, but reach beyond their petty plans and envision world peace and true Universal brotherhood. We must strive for a world unified in the truth that we are all part of God the Creator, operating from a state of cooperation and compassion rather than competition, domination and exploitation of others.

As spirituality becomes introduced into every aspect of human life, many societal institutions will crumble. Government is one such example where the power has shifted from the individual to the organization. As individual citizens grow increasingly threatened by the government, their focus should be on rising above the private agendas being played out globally and concentrating all their efforts in becoming spiritually evolved and as independent of government as possible. Always seek the highest meaning of all things. Come from a place of awareness and not fear in your dealings with the government. Everything is in constant evolution, including the government. Hopefully, enough individuals will infiltrate this self serving institution and evolve it by working from within. These souls will know all spiritual beings are bound together by a common thread, the Divine Principle, which is directed by the Creator. Our forefathers understood the meaning of spirituality as illustrated by their decision to include the words "One Nation under God" within our Constitution.

As our nation moves into the new millennium this new breed of statesmen will show its brothers and sisters on other parts of the planet that government symbolizes an enormous body made up of two hundred and sixty million cells represent ing every citizen. It will move out of its present dis- eased state into the light of harmony and self governing principals moving in synchronicity with the Universal laws of God. Just as government needs to evolve, so does the institution of organized religion so that it may serve its original purpose.

CHAPTER 10
ORGANIZED RELIGION

According to Webster's Dictionary, religion is: the personal commitment to and serving God with worshipful devotion and conduct in accord with divine commands as declared by authoritative teachers. A religious group, sect, church, denomination or cult can be defined as the body of institutionalized expressions of sacred beliefs, observances and social practices formed within a given cultural content. It is interesting to note Mr. Webster's definition neglects to mention the individual's own innate ability to receive information directly from the Creator obviating the need to follow commands from other individuals. The history of any religion contains three components: devotion, philosophy, and politics. Let us start with devotion.

Devotion, a truly spiritual act, is the earnestness and zeal in the performance of religious duties and observations carried out with religious fervor, reverence and piety to God. This can simply be expressed in an act of prayer or supplication. A devotee shows the highest degree of fidelity toward a supreme being. Regardless of how, when, where, or to whom, the act of devotion is a very holy and beautiful thing. To watch devotees perform remembrance to God is a truly moving experience. This special time may take the form of prayer, silence, meditation, contemplation, ritual or acts of devotion. Even within the framework of organized religion, you can easily identify those members who have made a decision to live a life of service to others and witness how their devotion carries them on a path toward the Creator. Devotion is an important and beautiful element of organized religion. Many individuals have taken this aspect of devotion and worked within organized religion to achieve truly exalted states. Saint Francis has shown to the world how to see God in all living creatures. Devotion has been practiced universally since the beginning of recorded time. Within any devotional practice lies a basic philosophical foundation.

The principles, theories, systems or rules that a particular religious order is based on is the philosophy of that religion. These philosophies are things of beauty and are integrated into the many traditions, teachings and beliefs adopted by the founder(s). Many religious philosophies are beautiful pieces of work: God is love, God is in all things, etc. The philosophy of religion, any religion, is also something to be admired. It is as spiritual as the devotion of the practitioners who believe in it and practice it. The philosophy to love your neighbor, mixed with the pursuit of wisdom and the quest for truth realigns you to your spiritual origins.

The last component of religion is politics. This omnipresent aspect of religion is far removed from any religious philosophy. History books are filled with information regarding the politics of religion and how throughout the evolution of the human species more lives have been lost in the name of religion than all wars put together. Since the beginning of time humans have been systematically exterminating each other for the sake of religion. During the Dark Ages to possess psychic abilities was considered heresy, the Devil's work, and the individuals were usually put to death. Why? Why is it that in the one place where love and peace are preached, you find more violence, hatred, bigotry, domination and death than in any other institution known to humankind? Unfortunately the motivation for many religious leaders changes with the acquisition of money and power. From that point on their message is guided by a private agenda masked as words from the Lord God.

When you hear such dichotomies as "God is love", and "God is All", but not you, or terms like sinner, repentance and unworthiness, take a step back and look closely. Have you ever wondered where you came from? What you were doing before you were born? How is it that you have no recollection of your previous state?

Where do you go when you die? The Church says heaven, well what is heaven? The church says wait and you'll find out. Why are so many questions left unanswered? Is it wrong to want answers? To want to know where you come from and where you go after this life? To the great masses of souls around the planet who have been indoctrinated for centuries, the word of God only reaches their ears through the spoken words of individuals who identify themselves as servants of the Lord or are ordained or affiliated with some religious organization. The reason for this originates from the belief that the people were so unintelligent and incapable of understanding the word of God that they had to be told what it all meant so that they could then understand.

Can you see the potential abuses of this system? Many religious sects, consider it a sin to read other religion's printed materials or to listen to other religion's belief systems. Why would this be? In many religions the very idea of God speaking directly through an ordinary person is heresy. Historically, Joan of Arc and many others were killed for proclaiming a direct connection to the Creator. Why? The answer is because religion is political and designed to control the masses. If you can form your own relationship with God then why do you need to support the elaborate hierarchy of a church, temple, or synagogue? Too often without even realizing it you demote and limit the infiniteness of the Creator to only being present in a single house of worship on a particular day of the week (Saturday or Sunday) and only speaking through someone outside yourself. Most every one was raised in one religion or another. In that religion you most likely were taught many of the beautiful philosophies such as love thy neighbor, God is love and the power of forgiveness. You may have learned about and developed sacred relationships with great teachers such as the Christ, Buddha, Mohammed, Moses and many others. Religion is important only in that it represents your starting point. It reminds you to stay tuned in to God.

In the Western culture, religions are generally conducted by religious leaders (usually males), preaching or reciting holy documents every Saturday or Sunday while their congregation passively listens to these words of purported wisdom and truth. The original purpose of religion was to help people evolve spiritually; to provide teachers for the purpose of leading others along their spiritual path. Perhaps the only true way to ensure you are evolving and not passively accepting beliefs of those institutions to which you affiliate yourself, is to constantly forge your own unique relationship with the Creator. You do this by praying or meditating on a regular basis. Rather than passively accepting the teachings and beliefs handed down to you, seek out your own truth.

Naturally religious groups make it easier by laying out a plan to follow instead of you pondering the truths of the Universe on your own. Although it is easier to follow a trodden path, the drawback is you end up with someone else's interpretation of the truth. Religion professes to intimately address the survival of the individual's spiritual evolvement by drawing on the zeal of many followers, but when these ideals become tyrannies, the means will always be justified by those professing the achievement of the altruistic goal. The misconceptions and the incorrect thinking taught by religion do not necessarily help humankind to find and stay on their spiritual path. Instead of religion freeing the soul of the individual, it keeps the soul locked into the belief system of that particular group and thus trapped in the Wheel of Karma. Without the focus of spiritually exalted goals using nonpolitical means, religion oppresses the very souls it was instituted to guide and support in spiritual unfoldment. This brain washing process has been in existence for so long that it is almost unthinkable to imagine you are born with all the tools it takes to be in continuous contact with your Creator. It is mainly through your sense of intuition that this link is made. Few religious orders, if any, acknowledge this natural innate ability in all human beings. When it is said: "God is all and God is everywhere," that also means you. You are all part of God! Unfortunately, the message usually heard includes such misconceptions as you are sinners and imperfect beings unworthy to receive God unless you repent for your sins.

The truth is you are born worthy to receive Grace from God. Even before you were born, you were capable of allowing the Divine Principle to flow through you. This Divine Creation is a matrix composed of minute particles directed by the Creator that binds everything together that exists within the Universe. This Divine Matter will flow through your soul and nourish all four of your natures. It is only when you feel unworthy and accept the erroneous messages from religious politicians that you feel separation from God. At that precise moment you accept your separateness from the Divine and unhappiness seeps into every cell within your body.

Sin is nothing more than incorrect thinking! Believing, for example, that you can harm another soul without karmic consequences is sinful. To steal from your neighbor and likewise believe you will not feel any repercussion is sinful. Lacking respect for self and others is sinful. Believing you can act dishonestly in your dealings with others and not be held accountable is sinful. These are all illustrations of incorrect thinking. You are born to experience harmony in the human condition, to learn whatever lessons you need to complete for the total unfoldment of your soul and thus escape the Wheel of Karma.

Few Western religious groups will acknowledge reincarnation. It is easy to see why this reality is kept secret and any reference to it removed from the Bible, since fear of Hell is what keeps parishioners coming back for more and congregations financially sound. Fear of eternal damnation is what motivates millions of worshipers toward religious dogma and away from their true greatness. If the phenomenon of reincarnation were as readily accepted as the existence of the Garden of Eden, people would clearly realize the importance of tidying up whatever loose ends they still have to resolve in order to return to the Oneness from whence they came. All paths lead Home, the place where all souls eventually come once they have become God realized! Whether you accomplish your mission in a single lifetime or 500,000 lifetimes, all souls now incarnated and even those who are not will eventually end up in the same place—Home, and thus doing so free themselves from the veil of ignorance and the Karmic Wheel.

A metaphor to explain this rather complex phenomenon is to imagine an infinite number of springs, each one representing an individual soul, being pulled in different directions from a single source. No two separate springs are known to have identical trajectories. The tension in each spring may be different, depending on how far it has traveled from its anchor. The anchor symbolizes Home, our Creator. No matter how much tension is present in each spring, representing lifetimes, in the end all springs must return to the anchor. All souls, the springs, have a single source. . . God. The Wheel of Karma can be thought of as the amount of resistance each spring faces in returning back to the anchor. To explain this concept you can imagine a magnet pulling each spring away from its source. The magnetic force the spring faces is determined by the attraction the spring has to its own magnet. This magnetic attraction can be thought of as your attachment to the physical world. In other words, the more attached you are to the physical world, the harder it will become for you to go Home. The Wheel of Karma is as real as gravity itself. The fact is the two phenomena are intimately related. To illustrate this connection imagine a soul traveling freely through the cosmos. For some reason, perhaps curiosity, it descends in vibrational frequency to add to its wisdom. By slowing down the rate at which its atoms spin, it eventually comes under the effect of a planetary electromagnetic field which exists in a three dimensional Universe. When finished, it must then gather enough power to jettison itself out of the gravitational pull of the planet, much the same way a rocket musters enough fire power to catapult itself into the limitless reaches of space.

Through the birth process the soul then enters the physical realm to experience sensory input and satisfy its needs. Depending on the soul's unique agenda while incarnated, it may not be possible for it to leave the planet's gravitational influence because of the accumulation of karma (attachment to the physical world) that must be repaid through other life times until the state of karmic neutrality is reached. At that point gravity will no longer have an effect on the soul (Wheel of Karma) and the soul can begin packing enough power to free itself to continue its journey through the cosmos in the mode of self discovery.

It is only through reaching true illumination, by escaping the grasp of karma and becoming God-realized, that you will truly know who you are. You will know from whence you came and understand your purpose in this life and where you are going. No longer will you need to die and forget all that you are. The veil of ignorance will be removed so that you may see the truth. Does organized religion help you reach this goal or does it perpetuate the veil of ignorance?

Organized religion reached its lowest point and stopped being synonymous with spiritual unfoldment during the Dark Ages. Gradually over the centuries, the mysteries of creation and life itself were lost in the hands of a few individuals within the higher ranks of the Church. For the sake of power and control over the masses, this knowledge was kept hidden from the people by the same individuals entrusted to teach it. Extraordinary experiences such as journeys out of body, raising of the Kundalini energy through the Chakras, levitation, teleportation, transmutation of the physical body and so on were censored from the masses. These are but glimpses of what the human species is capable of doing. You are indeed multidimensional beings, more than your physical bodies.

The physical body is made up of the basic building blocks of physical matter: the atom. Physical matter is less solid and much more etheric than it appears. It is but an illusion of the Light and Shadow your body houses. Atoms consist almost entirely of empty space. An atom is made up of three main components: protons, neutrons and electrons. The protons and neutrons are joined together to form the nucleus or core of the atom. Electrons orbit the nucleus at tremendous speeds. All of this is held together by an electromagnetic force. Matter is simply condensed forms (determined by the number of electrons and protons) of energy. Your physical body is a light body of matter in motion!

It was not possible for me to reconcile many of the lessons I (Peter), was taught as a child, raised Catholic, with the deeper understanding of myself and the glimpses of other realities that are also part of the Cosmos which I later experienced. Perhaps more so than in any other religion, the Catholic Church (being one of the largest of all organized religions) depicts the clearest example of misused power. Although it had a glorious be-ginning through our brother and teacher, Christ, the Church has long been converted into a global religio-political party. Examples which illustrate this major shift in philosophical teachings include celibacy, poverty and contraception. Christ never said, for example, celibacy is a requirement to become a spiritual counselor of the Church. To force an individual to remain without the physical love of another member of the same species is to suppress the natural experience of the soul. This unnatural state of being, forced upon the clergy by religious dogma, has led to a number of priests manifesting behavior not generally accepted by most societies. When I lived in the mountains of New Mexico, I witnessed everyday, numerous priests who had "gone astray" and had come to the mountains to reconnect. These poor priests included alcoholics, adulators, and pedophiles who were taken from their posts to be re-indoctrinated because they could not function under such strict rules.

Christ never said, poverty was the key to entering Heaven. There is absolutely nothing wrong with experiencing abundance. Wealth means abundance. Abundance is our natural state. Greed must not be confused with abundance. The camel through the eye of the needle parable was in reference to greed, not abundance. Many individuals have come to accept greed and abundance as synonymous conditions since that is the message they hear from religious leaders. Misconception and sinful interpretations of the original teachings given to us by Christ, are what has led to the present condition of the Catholic Church. Christ has been promoted as a beggar, which has been one of the greatest misconceptions of all time. Christ was not a poor man. Even the same church which tells us Christ was a beggar, recounts annually the Christmas story of three kings traveling great distances to bring gold, and offering their kingdoms to the Christ child. Why then is the belief that Christ was a beggar so largely propagated? In third world countries large populations are struggling to eat but they are sent the message that poverty is holy and that they will reap their rewards in the life to come. Consequently, millions of children perish each year from starvation. Tithing ten percent of ones income has become a policy of many religious groups. Why not instead tithe ten percent of your time to be with the Creator in prayer or meditation?

The Pope preaches that the responsible use of contraceptive devices, sterilization and even elective termination of a pregnancy are sinful acts. Regrettably, because of this inflexible stance on such an important issue, millions of women are giving birth to children whom they cannot even feed. The organizational pyramid of the church places enormous power on the shoulders of a single male, the Pope, who persists in holding onto an outmoded and unnatural position by banning the liberal use of birth control, enforcing celibacy among priests and preaching that poverty is the key to entering heaven. There are tremendous karmic repercussions to anyone who leads large numbers of people astray. To abuse your power and stop others from exercising their full range of expression is indeed sinful.*[1]

A good example of misuse of power is seen in Latin America where the overwhelming majority of citizens are Catholic. The Catholic Church is still very powerful in that part of the world and fear of God is the prevailing message many of those souls still hear. Control through fear and personal guilt is how the great masses of Latinos are coerced into believing being poor is a blissful and Godly state in which to live. They believe that to accept what the priest

---

1   *This was written in 1996 Agendas have changed.*

says without question is the only way to avoid the manmade concept of Hell. This is what happens when individuals relinquish their own power to others.

I (Elizabeth), recall a conversation I had one Christmas day in Martha's Vineyard with a scientist who said he did not believe in the Church because they expected you to have blind faith and he, being a scientist, needed proof before accepting anything as fact. I told him faith is important to tide you over until your consciousness has expanded enough to know something with certainty. One thing is for certain you were not intended to be complacent with blind faith. You must question and always strive to learn and grow. The problem for too long has been that science and spirituality have been separated. The truth is that the more you learn about spiritual phenomena, the more you learn about science. The true Bible and other spiritual books were scientific in nature. Much of their writings which are thought to be apocalyptic were misconstrued detailed steps in how to transmute the physical body. To understand the highest meaning of these religious books you must read them intuitively. Too often we become lost in the words and dialogue of these books never transcending our consciousness to achieve the exalted states to which these books refer. You must go beyond intellectually analyzing the words and merge with the book's vibration extracting the highest spiritual meaning.

Science has also proven to us that there are forces and energies that exist in the Universe that your senses cannot perceive. It has been scientifically documented that there exists a wide range of colors that the human eye cannot perceive. With the use of a special camera it can now be documented that living beings emit a certain life energy or aura which can now be photographed. It's amazing how many pictures the Hubble spacecraft has taken and many of the top scientists in the world have dissected the pictures and still come up with the same conclusion: there is no other intelligent life in the Universe. What do they expect it to look like? Rush hour traffic in L. A.? The problem is they do not know what they are looking at.

As you evolve your consciousness you move beyond the limits of form, you realize the most powerful life forces in the Universe are pure energies and not made up of physical matter as we know it. (Also, not all civilizations inhabit a planet's surface.) Based on simple logic it is arrogant and preposterous to believe humans are the only "intelligent" life in the entire Universe. All you need to do to prove this point is step outside one clear evening and spend about fifteen minutes silently observing the fiery stars and orbiting planets and other celestial bodies and humble yourself to the magnitude of this Universe. You will then come to the conclusion that there must be other intelligent life besides us, and they must have visited/visit planet Earth. One mistake many people make is that they believe any extraterrestrials or beings from another planet or dimension are holy and therefore to be worshiped. It is important to realize you are part of God and just as holy as these other creatures albeit some may have more awareness than you but you should not be in awe of them or taken in by any being just because they are not from here. It is a fact of life that when you travel abroad not everyone you meet is honest or trustworthy, so too the same rule applies to celestial beings who visit Earth. Some may be very evolved and others may not.

It would seem logical to assume technologically advanced extraterrestrials have visited the Earth before and influenced our history. Even the Bible and countless other religious documents refer to Chariots of Fire, wheels within wheels, etc. Mythology of various cultures including Greece talk of "the Gods" and other passages refer to messengers from God. Who were these "Gods?" Even Genesis opens by stating "The Sons of God married daughters of men." Is this a reference to the inbreeding that took place between extraterrestrials and indigenous humans long ago? Unfortunately, the Bible has been so tampered with by religious politicians that little of the truth remains. But one question I will ask: why is it that the Dead Sea Scrolls are protected by one of the most sophisticated security systems on the planet and remain unavailable to the masses? What are the world's religio-political leaders afraid of us learning? It has come time for you to grow up, to stop behaving like little children in dealing with organized religious leaders, seeing and hearing only what they want you to. Just as you must exercise self responsibility in the way you behave in every aspect of your life, this is especially true in matters of spiritual growth where you must be constantly on the alert for other people's agendas. In this delicate area you must not let someone else dictate how, when or if the Creator will communicate with you. Everyone has a teacher. It is your responsibility to decide what lessons you are ready to learn and from whom. This is your time to awaken. Religion is not spirituality. The highest spiritual level religion can achieve is to allow its practitioners the full expression of their intuitive powers. Everyone is a part of God. God lives within every cell in your body. Whether your priest, minister, pastor or rabbi agrees with you or not, you are a perfect living manifestation of God. Learn to appreciate the beauty of all things. Learn to respect all living creatures. God lives everywhere including inside yourself. It only takes a moment of thought to realize there is no such thing as a Baptist, a Mormon, a born-again Christian, a Catholic, a Hindu, a Jew or whatever.

Recently, I (Peter) saw a young patient distraught because her boyfriend broke off the relationship for no apparent reason. When she insisted for a reason he replied "Well, the fact is that we have no future together since I am a Baptist and you are a Mormon." Religions are man made subdivisions of the same thing. You are all brothers and sisters. The same Divine Principle flows through each and every one of you. This also applies to our celestial friends. We must not blindly follow any person or being just because they possess greater technology or can do neat tricks. The time has come for us to take responsibility for the direction of our planet. It is precisely because so many of you have bought into those labels that human suffering has been around for so long.

The simple truth is you are all members of the same species with various skin colors, height and weight, and live on various land masses of the same planet or off planet. Organized religion and other predominately male dominated institutions will have you believe differently. Governments, corporations, social groups and even schools will preach to their members that they are somehow better than other similar groups. That is simply not true. History books are full of tragic examples of what happens when a race of humans come to believe they are superior to another. The truth is you are all chosen and equal in the eyes of God. You are all chosen to receive grace from God. A moment of contemplation will reveal to anyone the constant indoctrination that goes on at all levels in our society. The sooner you realize this fact, the faster you will begin to live and function at the spiritual level you are meant to. Accepting as absolute truths the messages most religious orders give today is what will keep you trapped in the Wheel of Karma, incarnating time and time again.

Contrary to what organized religion teaches, living a life full of personal sacrifices, shying away from abundance and donating your wealth to the church rather than tithing your time to be with God is not your goal. Going through the death process as good Christians and reaching heaven is likewise not even remotely the spiritual level you want to achieve. It is amazing so many intelligent people subscribe to the JudoChristian belief that if you are a "good" Christian, Jew, etc., when you die you will go to "heaven," a place for nice people. Perhaps you are familiar with the story of the Buddha. According to the story, Buddha lived a good life and so when he passed from this plane he went to heaven. After spending an infinite amount of time doing whatever his heart desired, he asked the authorities there, "Isn't there more?" and so he came back, reincarnated and became Buddha the Christ. He escaped the Wheel of Karma which is nothing more than a guiding light on a blind ally. Buddha showed others how to get off the merrygoround. The best example of "heaven" is in the Star Trek movie, "New Generations," where Captain Kirk gets stuck in the Nexus. Captain Picard finds him indulging in all his desires. Picard then helps Kirk to awaken to the realization that he is living an illusion. At that point he decides to leave the Nexus, go back and "make a difference." Many of you long to make a difference, to become real players in the Great Plan and escape the web of illusion.

We realize in these shifting times when so much is being churned up and many of you feel confused, it is normal to flock to the comfort of "old time religion." I (Elizabeth), was speaking to my mother the other day and she recounted how her own mother had been put into a nursing home recently and was having a hard time dealing with the situation. Apparently during a visit to the nursing home, they started playing some hymns. Both she and her mother began to sing and soon tears filled their eyes. While the familiarity of religion can be temporarily comforting, the question to ask is: Is your religion taking you where you want to go, or are you becoming like so many old folks who crowd the pews every Sunday morning holding onto what is familiar while their bodies and minds grow old and feeble? Is the religious practice you are currently engaged in taking your further along your pathway towards God realization? Are you getting off the Karmic Wheel, leaving dis- ease behind?

Almost every belief that holds you back and gets in the way of reaching Godrealization comes from some religious belief. Even if you had no religious upbringing, or you feel you are not bound by the beliefs of the faith you practiced or were raised in. I invite you to review your day as detached as possible and examine your reactions and decisions. A very Christian belief is to suffer and work hard in this lifetime reaping your rewards in the life hereafter, putting one more star in your halo every time you delay your reward. How many times do you fail to allow yourself to collect the rewards life offers you? How many times do you continue in your present pain and emotional turmoil somehow believing it will get better tomorrow? The notion that everything will be okay when you die may sound silly but billions of souls accept that theory without conscious awareness. This belief is completely illogical. For example, if your check book does not balance today, tomorrow it is not going to magically balance unless you find out what went wrong. The same is true for the student who has not studied for a test and yet expects to know all the answers when the day of the exam arrives. The Judo Christian religions teach that all your problems will miraculously be resolved when you die. The truth is this is not how the system works. Just as a reputable University will not grant you a degree until you pass all of the required courses, so too you must pass all of life's courses in order to graduate. So many well meaning individuals actually believe that when the time of death arrives they will be absolved from all their problems and "go to rest" in a place called heaven. As it has previously been mentioned, there is no death, only a change of form. Therefore, after death you find yourself without a physical body but with the same set of problems. After a "rest period" you get the opportunity to come back with no memory and do it again, hopefully right this time. I recall in "Zorba the Greek," the main character became angered at the priest's lack of knowledge and asked, "What's the good of all your books if you can't explain why things happen?" Western religion can never have these answers because they are only looking at the tip of the iceberg. Since reincarnation has been removed from the Bible, there is no way to explain why people are born with physical or emotional obstacles or handicaps.

One afternoon we were having lunch at a food court in Palm Springs, California and we shared a table with an attractive older woman. This individual noticed we took a moment of silence to give thanks for the nourishment we were about to receive. After we finished praying she asked what church we attended and I (Elizabeth), replied "We don't do organized religion." She asked why and I told her I didn't find my answers there. She remarked, "well, nobody has all the answers." Her remark was quite profound and truthful. Nobody has all the answers, except the Creator. There will always be questions and answers as you remain in the mode of self discovery. I have found many answers to my questions, but few came from organized religion.

Learning to resonate your physical body at the highest possible frequency to receive as much Light as you can is a realistic goal many of you can reach in this lifetime. You do this by purifying all four of your natures and then begin to resonate from a place void of any karma in alignment with God's Will and your divine purpose. At this point you can truly begin to function as a Christ being of God.

It is important to appreciate the true meaning of the word Christ which is a specific level of consciousness achievable by anyone who dedicates himself/herself to God without reservation. For example, Jesus (a) the Christ, Buddha the Christ, Muhammad the Christ, and so on. Think of it as an office or a position which carries with it authority and a great deal of responsibility. The true Ascended Masters that have came before and after him, knew this fundamental truth. Christ is the door through which you must pass to return Home to the Creator, the same way the prodigal son returns home to his father. In this metaphor you represent the son and God, the Creator, represents the father. Unfortunately, somewhere along the way most Christian sects lost this information and so for centuries they have been preaching that you should stop at the threshold of the door. The end result is that many well meaning Christians have been worshiping the door rather than passing through it. To be worshiped is not why Christ incarnated. He came to preserve the truth and to be an example and to help us to be like him, not worship him.

One Christmas I (Elizabeth), was visiting with my family in Kentucky. The topic of Christ came up for discussion by the group of women which included an ordained minister. The question I raised to the group was why did Jesus come to this planet? When I voiced my opinion, which was to show us the way, many family members agreed, but felt they could not be like Christ, or obtain Christ consciousness in this lifetime. Since no one present at the table believed in reincarnation, it was impossible for them to imagine ever achieving this goal. If you cannot even entertain the idea that you could follow the example Jesus the Christ has set and be like him, then what was the purpose of his life here? Certainly, it may seem easier to worship someone than to start the difficult and disciplined task of following the example they set.

The many great teachers who have come to Earth are humble beings who do not need to feed their ego by demanding worship from others. Jesus is obviously not the only human to have ever ascended, although the Christian world seems to think he is the only son of God. The truth is we are all Sons of God. The truth is Buddha, Muhammad, Moses, Babaji, and many others have come before us and achieved the same level of awareness. They have all come, and will continue to do so, to make our pathway Home easier. As you enter the new millennium many of you will awaken and realize you are fully capable of reaching God-realization in this lifetime. Those who have gone before you, together with a host of other God-realized beings who are now with us, are extending their hands out to you in hopes that you will, at last, awaken from the dream, the illusion of the physical world, and take your rightful place living in accordance with God's Will and in harmony with your fellow brethren. This goal can only be achieved by following your life path, integrating your four natures into the four human activities.

Section Five:
The Four Activities

Proper balance in all four human activities hastens spiritual unfoldement.

CHAPTER 11
RELATIONSHIPS

There are only four activities a human engages in during the course of her/his daily. They are relationships, work/ education, playtime and devotion. If any one of these areas are dis- eased they will bleed into all other aspects of your life. Therefore it is of the greatest importance to attend to these areas and utilize correct thinking and correct action at all times.

Relationships are an important activity that everyone participates in, and probably represents the most challenging area of an individual's life. How do you live in harmony with those souls around you? How do you grow in your own unique direction and allow those around you to grow in theirs? How do you maintain intimacy and closeness, yet allow space for each other to grow? How can you see your partner as a playmate and cocreator, rather than a rival or persecutor? These are some of the questions that immediately arise when relationships are discussed.

One of the major problems on this planet is that nobody understands sex. The male's reproductive organ is exposed, while the female's are hidden. This symbolizes the way masculine energy works, exposed. There is no mystery to it. By contrast the feminine force is hidden. The original seed for the Universe was masculine and all other aspects of creation are feminine. This principle can best be explained by regarding the male of the species as the one who provides the seed and the female as the one who expands upon it. During the act of procreation the male gives forth sperm, the woman receives them and transforms the creation into an entire human being. Once the man has given forth the seed his job is finished, the feminine aspect must take over. It is easy to trace this principle back to tribal times when the man hunted and brought the prey back to the woman. She then cooked the meat for nourishment, cleaned the hide for clothing, used the bones for utensils and so on until every part of the animal found a useful purpose.

The feminine energy is the most powerful energy in the Universe! The feminine aspect is constantly reaching out for the new. Many males become fearful of this awesome power and suppress the feminine aspect within themselves and in the females around them. In most third world countries women are treated like beasts of burden while in this country one of the examples of female suppression goes under the name of "the right to life movement." Close scrutiny will reveal this movement is not about saving lives but domination of females. They seek to deny women the God given right to be masters of their own temples. It is unfortunate that the masculine force strives to control, enslave, and dominate the feminine aspect when the true function of the male is to care for, nurture and help the female to better know herself. When the male can properly love and support the female, then he can learn and grow from the wisdom and bountiful gifts the female so graciously offers him. The female in turn can encourage the dreamer in the male.

The male's function in lovemaking is to help the female open in her root chakra, then in her heart and in her mind. As she unfolds she is able to more freely express love, and can be more intuitive in seeing patterns in the family, community, country and in the Universe. By this unfoldment she can better serve humanity and thus everyone wins. The men win because if they can humble themselves and listen to the female, they can learn from her intuition and guidance. The women win because they receive love and nurturing from their partners.

The woman's job is to steer and direct the male in a gentle and loving way. If the woman can do this from a loving position, and the men can set aside their fears and listen, this planet may find a way out of its present dilemma. True power lies in one's softness. We have three dogs. Our two male dogs are always competing with each other, trying to see who can pee higher up on a tree. Princess, our female dog, is always looking around to see if anyone needs her while she squats to pee. Their behavior symbolizes the cooperative nature in females and the competitive nature in males. Little boys, like our dogs, are always trying to show mom how high up on the tank they can pee, how far they can throw, or how high they can jump. By comparison, little girls are always helping their mothers, taking care of dolls and/ or baby brothers or sisters. The time has come for the men to start squatting and looking around to see who needs them and how they can be of service to others and for the women to start seeing how high they can jump.

In my counseling I (Elizabeth), see women who have lost touch with their own power. These individuals are afraid to break out and try their own wings. Instead they end up taking care of everyone else but themselves. Charity begins at home! You come first, then it spreads to your mate, then to your children, then to your community and so forth. Contrary to this principle, women take care of everyone else, except themselves, thus failing to make others responsible for their own actions. Self esteem and self worth need to be reprogrammed into the minds of women. The image of a "good Christian woman" is so stifling there is very little room for self power or creative expression. Women must reconnect with that powerful creative force within them which moves them and nurtures them. There is nothing evil about the female's natural intuitive and expressive abilities. It is in the cooperative, creative and intuitive aspect of a woman that the true power lies!

Men and women possess both masculine and feminine energies. Hormonally men make estrogen (the main female hormone) and women make testosterone (the principal male hormone). Innately, men have the powerful female energy within them. Regrettably society continues to separate, segregate and strip away the human's harmonious nature. Gender roles are so ingrained into every culture that it takes a conscious effort to grow out of them. As a youngster I (Peter), recall having lots of opportunities to learn to play the piano. Peer pressure, however, convinced me that I should play another instrument because the piano was considered "too feminine." Sadly this is what many males are confronted with throughout their development. Proverbs such as "Boys will be boys" encourage this aberrant type of behavior for the human species. Men grow up believing it is not normal or socially acceptable to be sensitive. Women are molded into submissive creatures taught that they are incapable of functioning as a whole individual without a man's support.

Imagine two toddlers playing together in a sandpile. A boy and girl are playing together, exploring and learning about each other. They are best friends and playmates. At this point in their lives there is no gender difference. As they build their own sand castles they are free to go wherever their imagination leads them. The moment these two toddlers enter the school system, the first thing that happens is that they learn separation and segregation of the sexes: Boys to the right and girls to the left. When the same couple grow up and become teenagers, the whole gender mind set is imprinted. By this time they have lost the innocence of being "best friends" and in-stead have become rivals. Both individuals are forced to meet an entirely different code of expectations taught to them by a society that does not understand sex.

How many times have you females, lamented about your relationship stating "the problem is he is not sensitive enough?" If all humans have both masculine and feminine qualities, why aren't men more sensitive? The answer is simple—women did not want sensitive men, they wanted providers. So men evolved into slick, quick and strong creatures able to win the prize. Think about it for a moment.

Women all dolled up and hung on their man's arm just like a prize won at a carnival as if she were a trophy for his being the slickest, quickest and strongest. Attributes such as gentleness, softness and a greater ability to express love are left to the female gender. This fundamental misconception transcends into every aspect of your life. Therefore it is easy to see why societal institutions function under the premise: man rules, woman obeys.

Another grave misperception that is ingrained in so many cultures is that the male is the king of the castle. He is the head of the household, the one who wears the pants. Man orders, woman serves. I (Elizabeth), caught a few moments of a talk show where they interviewed women who felt their husbands treated them like slaves. The truth is everyone loses because of this great misperception of things. The men may appear to be the top dog but are in fact fearful and inflexible. Yousee this pattern in couples who grow old together where the wife often has an underlying resentment toward her husband which she has harbored for years. She denies her husband sex and/or hates the entire experience. As he grows old and softens, he longs for his wife's love and attention, but by this time she is emotionally unavailable. Usually these men die of heart attacks, alcoholism, or are crippled with arthritis.

Frequently in households where men are rigid and inflexible, they can be easily manipulated because true power belongs to the one who is soft. Like the firm and unmovable rock which is worn down in time by the constant movement of a river, so have women become masters at wearing men down. This is precisely where the problem lies and ultimately leads to a breakdown of all communication. Partners can no longer have a relationship or even a conversation for free. Unless a level of communication is reached where the female can openly express her desires and opinions, she will continue to manipulate her partner into doing what she wants. As a result, the male does everything in his power to avoid contact with the female. Consequently, the men go out with the guys and the women congregate with the girls. With time you forget the reason you came together in the first place which was to be best friends and playmates!

Any relationship can be a real challenge. A daughter's relationship with her father or a son's relationship with his mother is substantially different than a mother/daughter relationship, or a father/son relationship. How would you feel as a little person if your mother (if you are a man) or your father (if you are a woman) were to leave you? That is the same feeling you have about your partner, fear of abandonment! At certain moments in the relationship one member may seem to have the upper hand and says, "I don't need you anymore, I"m leaving!" "No, don't go!" cries the other. But the truth is both partners are afraid of abandonment. Unfortunately, the illusion of one upmanship continues and as you become competitors rather than playmates the relationship begins to suffer. "I've got him wrapped around my little finger" boasts one partner or "She worships the ground I walk on" replies the other. How many times have you heard or said these words which indicate competition? And the battle of the sexes rages on.

You must call a truce and learn to move as one. You must realize when you abuse the person sitting across from you physically, mentally, emotionally or spiritually, you are in fact abusing yourself. Part of the human journey is to bring the masculine and feminine energies into balance. These Yin and Yang energies can be blended and harmonized through the power of love. Part of the female's role is to educate and guide the male with love and softness, but first she must blend with the male's energy accepting his lower vibration which harmonizes and balances her own higher vibration. If the female does not blend or merge with the male, the male will outshine the female and her energy will shatter. As a gynecologist I (Peter), have seen countless cases of women who have problems ranging from breast dis- ease to uterine cancers. These are manifestations of the powerful female energy which has not been balanced by male energy. The male's job, on the other hand, is to romance the female. He seeks out the female's light. The female must then accept the male's energy, thus merging with the male and balancing out her own energy. One of the most important ways the female can blend with the male and accept his seed, but not the only way, is through the act of lovemaking.

Love making is one of the most spiritual activities an individual could possibly partake in. Unfortunately, women have been handed a truckload of beliefs which foster denial of their femininity and sexual desires. As a way of merging with the masculine energy women need to accept their sexuality and allow themselves to be fully aroused by their male partners. They need to completely participate in the sexual act and allow themselves to become open in their sexual organs, in their hearts, in their minds, and in their spirit. The male's role is to help the female unfold. The male must express his love in a gentle and sensitive way, being fully aware of his partner's needs and desires. Sexuality, in particular the orgasmic experience, is a moment of ecstasy that nurtures all four of your natures simultaneously. It is a brief reminder that you are a creature of God. What does an orgasm mean to you? A goal? Something sinful? Something that happens to other people but not you? You all have the capacity to feel this wonderful experience as often as you like, with someone or alone. It is insecurities, incorrect thinking, and the inability to relax that stops you from enjoying such moments. Humans are all meant to be orgasmic beings.

You are designed to feel God's presence through the Kundalini arousal initiated by lovemaking. Regrettably, organized religion has tainted the act of love making into something sinful. The foundation for this is that sex is synonymous with lust. As you evolve spiritually it is correct and natural for your Kundalini energy to be aroused. It is helpful to your evolvement to activate this energy frequently. The mistake that often occurs is that the individual chooses to draw in other sexual partners instead of confining his/her activities to his/her mate, or if you are single the activity of hoping from one partner to the next. This creates stress and causes you to lose your original focus of union with God. Not only does this create disharmony and dis- ease emotionally and mentally, but physically as well. As a gynecologist I (Peter) see the results of this action in the form of multiple communicable dis- eases, AIDS being one of the most devastating. To those of you engaging in sex with multiple partners, I say this: you can know the entire ocean by knowing a single drop. For those engaging in multiple sexual encounters, I recommend buying something battery operated which is more convenient and much safer.

As your relationship with your partner grows, the complete and freely given exploration and sharing of your physical temple in a gentle, loving way, becomes a beautiful and natural act which is integrated into your life together. Through this holy act of sharing the seed is planted by the male into the female. The egg, symbol of femininity, is thus fertilized and from this union grows a whole human being. A truly incredible event of God manifesting God that has lost its extraordinary significance because it happens so often. What a wonderful living proof of God. As an obstetrician, I have been fortunate to witness the birth of these divine creations over 3,500 times and it still awes and amazes me at the perfection of this process.

Parenting your offsprings through their apprenticeship until they are ready to leave you and continue on their own path then becomes the natural order of things. Regrettably, so many people rush into parenthood for the wrong reasons. Many young women, lacking warmth and nurturing at home, seek companionship from the opposite sex. They find themselves pregnant and wanting to have a baby so that they will have someone to love them. I (Elizabeth), believe that people should start having children when they fill truly ready. This way they can give themselves enough time to learn from life's experiences. This business about a biological clock has caused more anxiety over an event that is about love and self discovery, not time tables. Give you and your partner time to get to know each other and to act as playmates before the responsibilities start to stack up.

A question to contemplate which depicts the true meaning of an intimate relationship is this: It's the middle of the night. There is a fire in your house! You awaken and realize there is only enough time to save yourself and one other member of your family. Who would you choose? Your spouse or one of your children? The answer is your playmate.

Your function as parents is to help your children discover their own power, make choices, learn self responsibility and encourage self love, respect for their physical temples, and all life forms including Mother Earth. Help your children develop a strong self image, to know where their talents, gifts and abilities lie. Teach them to appreciate their own greatness with humility as "sparkles of God" on this planet, and set examples for them in the giving and receiving of love. When we are born, we come into the world through the birth canal. We choose our parents for body type, old business and new business. Parents are one of the courses we take on planet Earth to learn more about ourselves. (Like skin color, geographical location, and social economical status). We apprentice under our parents to learn a way of being. Then we become journeymen, and go out to learn our own way of being in the world until we can become Masters. That's it! Parents are just there to teach us a way to be in the world until we are old enough to start discovering our own way.

Unfortunately, parents lacking their own sense of self esteem and self worth foster dependency in their children and rob them of their God given right of self discovery, independence, and right to find their own power. When a woman is lacking a supportive and nurturing relationship with a male, and she has a male child, that child often becomes her relationship. This act of what Italians call *mammismo* robs the male from ever gaining a sense of his own power. He grows up emotionally plugged onto his mother's breast. Because of this, he is unable to be there for his mate in a loving and supportive way and so the cycle of emotional dependency upon the mother figure is perpetuated.

As the only child born to a very domineering maternal figure, I (Peter), realized the harmful effects my strong bond with my mother had on my relationships with members of the opposite sex. Physically distancing myself from my mother helped me to evolve beyond her. Over the years the relationship has evolved to a level where both my mother and I can enjoy each other's company. In other words, the relationship is now free with no expectations being placed by either one of us.

As role models from which children learn to form references to the rest of the world, you need to establish boundaries. Children are like horses who when placed in a new pasture, circle the perimeter to find any holes or weak spots in the fence. Once they are satisfied there is no escape, they can relax and graze. Children are much the same way, they will always test their parents to find a hole in the boundaries. Often marital difficulties exist which keep the parents from acting as a unified front in the disciplining of their offsprings. The children are then triangulated into the dysfunctional marriage between the two parents and are unable to get on with their lives. The gift children bring to grown ups is exposing any and all holes or weak spots you may have. Once the child is satisfied there are no holes or weak spots, they can get down to the business of being a child.

Parenting is a tough job. You are not there to become your child's best friend. You are the parent! Your job is to make decisions about what is best for your children. Many parents are intimidated by their own children and are afraid to take charge and be the parent. You must set rules and boundaries to create and maintain safety, then give your children plenty of room for self discovery. Help them to know their unique talents and individual gifts. Your children are not there for you to fill an empty space in your life, nor are they there to follow in your footsteps or do the things you never had the courage to do. It is easy to become involved and interfere when you see your children engaged in activities you do not approve. Next time this happens you may want to ask yourself this question: Am I about to stop this activity solely for the purpose of exercising my power, or am I performing a duty as a parent untainted by my own beliefs?

Children are not yours to control and manipulate to fit your agenda, they are separate souls who have their own unique story. They are not there to live out your dreams or reach your expectations. In the octopus species the female conceives, then nests until her offspring is born. At that point she withers and dies. Many females consider themselves incomplete without their young ones always at an arms reach. Their sole purpose for living is to provide a safe haven for their children. In their world, other relationships come second to their role as mothers. Their roles as mates and their own needs and desires are squashed by the demands they place upon themselves as maternal figures to their offsprings. Like the octopus they begin to wither and die. For so long women have been taught to put their lives aside and build their world around their husband and children. This is incorrect thinking. When you live in this incorrect manner, you find yourself lowering your own selfesteem and lacking a strong self image. You become resentful of those around you. You cannot encourage independence and freedom in others if you do not encourage it in yourself. The only remedy to this incorrect thinking is to get a life! Start small, maybe take some classes in some form of creative expression, such as an art class or a dance class. Get that degree you always wanted. Start a new sport, the more active the better. Hire a baby sitter and give yourself sometime off. Go for walks on your own. Get your creative juices flowing! Reconnect with who you are. Take some risks. Start a business! You must come together with your mate and your children as an independent and selfreliant soul. Just as a tree cannot grow in the shadow of another, love cannot grow where there is dependency and attachment. "And

God created Adam and Eve," a pair, a couple. The number two symbolizing balance. The balancing of two energies which integrates both masculine and feminine qualities from each partner. A spiritual partnership therefore is the coming together of two separate and distinct souls for the purpose of learning life's lessons through the process of self discovery. As you learn about the giving and receiving of love, you both grow closer to the Creator. When you look into the eyes of your mate you see God staring back at you. A patient I (Peter), saw recently comes to mind in describing relationship conflicts. She was terrified of her husband who beat her on a regular basis. Her children cried frequently, apparently fearful of what was going on around them. Feeling trapped and yet unwilling to take the first step out of her misery she cried "but I still love him dearly." I concluded it was not my business to interfere but to give options.

If the relationship is not nurturing to both partners, as my patient illustrates, then the partner who is not being nurtured should ask him or herself this question: Why am I in this relationship? What am I suppose to learn from all of this? Frequently, the answer will pop into the individual's mind saying yes, stay here for there are still lessons to be learned. Other times the answer is no, it is over. Relationships do end. When the gifts have been given and there is no more to give, then, it is time to move on. This does not mean the relationship failed or you failed because it is over. Many couples swear to stay together "till death do us part." This means the death of the relationship, not the death of their physical bodies. Many couples decide to stay together "for the sake of the children." For the sake of the children move on and find your own happiness, be an example to them of how charity begins with yourself first. Remaining in a dysfunctional relationship does more harm to the children as the tension between the parents builds and a poor model of the giving and receiving of love is reinforced daily. Children will recover from a divorce and will have an opportunity to forge their own relationship with each parent, if the parents can be mature enough not to interfere. When the relationship ends, that particular avenue of self discovery has been fulfilled. In these cases it is best to end the relationship quickly. You need to cut it with a knife, not a butter knife. Often abusive situations result when one of the partners stays in the relationship too long. If your partner breaks up with you stop asking your self what is wrong with me, what did I do wrong? The answer is nothing! The gift has been given, your partner has nothing left to give you. You get what you need and move on. Hopefully, both partners can still appreciate the gift each of they received from their partner while the partnership lasted. No matter what factors lead to the breakup, even the most dysfunctional relationship offers a gift to the individual. If nothing else, it is the gift of finally realizing you do not want to have that kind of relationship any more.

Anger and hate too often serve as the fuel for dismantling the relationship and blocking your grief. The message usually heard from parents, friends, relatives and lawyers is that the other partner is responsible for what happened. The goal often then becomes financial security as the price paid by the former mate for abandoning the relationship. Most often the attorneys are the ones to gain the most from the discord that ensues. Why proceed along those lines?

Why not instead part as friends? People change. People grow. As old lessons are learned new ones are presented. Get what you need and move on. Each partner has a unique path to follow. What if the individual is between relationships? Not everyone needs to be in a relationship. Think of all the freedom you have. Enjoy that freedom! If you still want to get back into another relationship, then this time becomes a great opportunity to ask the Universe for the right partner. The next question then becomes, who is the right partner? One who has the capacity to give and receive love. Not every one can. One who has similar philosophies to yours. You do not want someone who thinks exactly the same as you do because that would be boring. Someone who you enjoy being with and s/he enjoys being with you in return. Someone you are physically attracted to and who is attracted to you. That is the definition of a perfect partner. Unlike what you may have heard, the perfect partner does not have to be your soul mate. You will notice such qualities as intelligence, financial status, height, weight, sex, color of skin, etc., are not included in the definition of a perfect partner! These issues may come up for most people since society has deemed them important. Don't allow social beliefs to stop you from enjoying the company of a partner for life.

Is a spiritual relationship synonymous to marriage? Although it is meant to be, often it is not. Have you heard the old saying, " it's a marriage of convenience," or "she married for money?" Frequently two people come together for the wrong reasons, expecting to receive something from the marriage. They approach the relationship with an ulterior motive counting on the other partner to provide money, position, security or even love. They may come together to control, dominate or abuse their partner. Partners may be looking for an accountant, a therapist, or a handy person. These are all the wrong reasons to come together. You come together to be playmates and best friends! As a loving and spiritual being you have the right to give and receive love. The free exchange of ideas, desires and the joy of observing another human being while evolving through life experiences is available to you. Sharing moments that fulfill you and your partner emotionally, physically, mentally and spiritually is the manner in which you were intended to relate to one and other. When a spiritual partnership has evolved to a certain point then the relationship is for free. You are then joined together in purpose and as playmates without expectations and attachments.

What if two males, or conversely two females, decide to form an emotional partnership? Does society have the right to eradicate that type of behavior? Are humans meant to be in a spiritual partnership only with members of the opposite sex? You all possess masculine and feminine qualities. Sometimes two men, for example, come together because their souls need to experience a unique type of energy expressed through an individual of the same gender. The same principle holds true for females in a relationship needing to experience the nurturing from another female who may be expressing a masculine quality through her personality. It is not up to society to decide what types of intimate relationships are acceptable and which are not, or to set rules regarding who an individual can love and who they cannot. Any partnership that nourishes both individuals in the four aspects of their being, regardless of gender, is the right relationship for the souls involved. A soul has no gender. A loving, nurturing intimate relationship between two members of the same sex, is as holy as one between two members of the opposite sex. In my own experience I (Peter), have seen many living examples of same sex relationships that were as loving as my own.

An intimate relationship is the best model to teach the individual whatever lessons s/he needs to learn in order to move forward toward Godrealization. It is easy to see why this is so, since often in the course of several years every conceivable issue will come up which can be applied to other relationships or activities outside the partnership. What better way to evolve socially than to learn how to truly love your partner and to be able to see the sparkle of the Creator in their eyes and know that God is looking back at you!

Another type of relationship which needs to be covered here is the one between you and your parents. As children, most every one clings to the fantasy that they can heal their parents. As a selfrealized adult, you can see your parents as separate souls following their own path and beliefs which are unique to them. You are not responsible for anyone else but yourself. The present relationship we have with our parents is one of love and honor. You can be a living example to your children, your parents, friends and spiritual partner. This does not mean you must sacrifice yourself in order to bring them happiness and joy. You must accept responsibility for your own growth which is first and foremost. The ability to give and receive love is the goal of any relationship, including the one with your parents. The current working model of a family relationship expects all members to intermingle in each other's story. When a member has a personal crisis, it often becomes the family's crisis. This type of behavior prevents each member from the freedom to fully express them selves. This is a common social error as, the fact is, all of us have unique and separate paths. Once you are able to develop sufficient awareness and intuitive skills to identify hidden messages, you can then effortlessly detach yourself from their influence and free yourself from familiar entanglements. Your relationship can then respect individual boundaries and encourage independent growth towards Godrealization. As you move out of dysfunctional relationships and behavior patterns you will free yourself to heal all areas of your life. As you are no longer distracted or pulled into destructive patterns with those around you a greater degree of self knowledge and self love can occur. You will then easily move into your higher purpose for incarnating on this planet at this time.

CHAPTER 12
WORK, EDUCATION, PLAYTIME, AND DEVOTION

The other three activities which occupy the rest of your time are work or education, playtime and devotion. Work often becomes the main activity to the exclusion the other three. In the American culture people generally become consumed by their jobs leaving little time for relationships, recreation and devotion. Workaholics are by products of those nursed by the Puritan work ethic and reared under the Industrial Revolution. Being a workaholic does not necessarily mean that you are more productive. On the contrary, often you become so drained by your excessive busyness, your creative energy becomes stifled leading to inflexibility and resistance to change.

The American culture places too much emphasis on your role as a worker. You are your job. People identify themselves according to what they do for a living. "I am a lawyer, a doctor or an accountant." Do you define yourself by your work? Do you think like a teacher, a doctor or an engineer? Is that the group of people with whom you most frequently socialize? Does your work mask who you really are? The letters you carry behind your name are irrelevant; what you learn about yourself in the process of your work is. The truth is, you are God wearing various hats to aid in your own self discovery. That's where the focus needs to be.

You are meant to have different and diverse jobs that feed all four of your natures. By performing different duties you are more likely to experience a greater variety of situations to help unfold your own life story. Fear of losing a pension, tenure, or financial status should not be a consideration. As you progress and learn from a particular job, management will provide another opportunity which will most likely be an upgrade. Financial abundance is always a part of this upgrade. As you learn to use faith to open doors while remaining unattached, a new job may present itself which is not exactly what you want. Take it! Once you are in the door and have learned your way around, the original job you sought may appear. An opportunity may present itself that is the opposite of what your ego wants, but will provide growth for your soul. Seize the opportunity you are directed towards and remember things aren't always what they seem. Management will never steer you wrong!

Another important aspect of work is service. Your job, no matter how small, affords you the opportunity to join in the hierarchy of beings (upper management) who have dedicated themselves to serve our planet and the Creator. No matter how mundane the task may seem, approach your job with devotion and a sense of craftsmanship realizing you are doing something important. The opinion of others should not be a consideration since you are not performing your duties to have your ego stroked by others. Perhaps dutifully doing your job may mean confronting powerful entities that exist in your community, city or country. You must have the courage to remain focused on your true purpose and not waste your time by pleasing the wrong people.

A few years we took a trip to Italy where I (Elizabeth), had lived for many years. While in Naples we visited a cameo factory and observed an old man carving a new piece. We were amazed at the patience and attention he showed to his craft. Slowly and meticulously he polished and molded each one with delicate care and precision. We noticed the same care and attention to detail exhibited by many workers in Italy. Each waiter took great pride and attention in his duties. Every cafe had an employee who strived to make the perfect cappuccino. Even cleaning the floor or washing the dishes was a duty taken very seriously and handled with skill and attention. By contrast, it has become apparent to many people in this country that craftsmanship is a quality noticeably lacking. Countless times you run into disgruntled employees whose focus is far removed from providing service. Mediocracy and incompetency run rampant in American society. You find yourself spending countless hours performing tasks that someone else should have done correctly in the first place. You must keep in mind that devotion should be present in every activity you undertake no matter how menial. Everything is spiritual! It is your ego that classifies a job as good or bad.

Creativity and a sense of self discovery are all but absent from the market place. Human beings often resemble robots performing tasks in a rote fashion. We need more creativity pumped into our industries. The movie industry was one example where creativity historically has managed flourishes beside prosperity but not anymore. Most financially successful people are entrepreneurs who had the creative sparkle to think in new categories and the vision and faith to carry their ideas out. If you have a business idea that you've been wanting to start, go out and do it! Remember, it's all about self discovery. Use your faith to open the doors and put a lot of juice behind it, don't allow fear to immobilize you thus becoming enslaved by your work.

Life purpose, is an area of great confusion and pain to many individuals. Career counseling has flourished as one of the most sought after services. How can you find out on your own what your life purpose is or, if still in school, what to study? The first notion to dismiss is the idea that you need to choose a single job for the rest of your life. The future is for those who can wear many hats and be active in many projects. You choose your biological parents or step parents to apprentice under for the skills they had which may relate to your own purpose. Their jobs, interests and/or hobbies are clues which you must decipher to establish your purpose in this lifetime. This is a developmental process which means you need to look at how your parents evolved. For example, when you were just born what do you remember your father doing for work and hobbies? Was he a car salesperson? Did he like to fix things in his spare time, rebuild engines? What do you remember you mother doing for work and hobbies? Was she a homemaker? Did she enjoy cooking and sewing? What were your interests as a small child? Did you play indoors or out? Did you make up games? Play with dolls? Race GoKarts? These are all clues to discerning your true purpose. Look at the various ages of your life. What were your social and educational interests in preschool, elementary school, junior high, and high school? Look for shifts of interests and areas where your interests and your parents interests intersect. Perhaps your father was an architect and your mother enjoyed gardening and as a child you built sand castles at the beach. You could design and build environmentally sound homes. The idea is to look at your apprenticeship and put together creative and expansive jobs for yourself. Find something to do that you love and get a nice paycheck. Work is an evolving creative fun activity which is meant to provide you with the opportunity of self expression, and give you plenty of energy back (money is energy in the stand by mode). The highest meaning of purpose is to fulfill your life's agenda in accordance with the Divine Will of the Creator. "Thine will be done on Earth as it is in heaven."

In the world of business, the problem is that most corporations do not understand the meaning of sex. Regrettably society has developed with most institutions dominated by males employing their masculine aspect to the exclusion of their innate feminine attributes. Many of these businesses are constantly introducing new products or services (masculine activity). Once the seed is given, the masculine activity is over and the feminine aspect must take over. The focus is now placed on service and caring for the employees the fact that a product is produced or a service is rendered is secondary. Visiting the lobby of a large corporation always reveals a receptionist as the first employee who comes in contact with potential customers. She is the most important person in that business. Her work ethics and attitude become of paramount importance as her energy intermingles with others. Unfortunately, when corporate heads get together, the receptionist is almost never invited. Work is about working together. You come together as a family learning how to relate to one another on a soul to soul level. Most often individuals do their jobs very well but fall short in the area of interpersonal relationships. That's where the real challenge comes. It's not about who can make the most money or sell the best product.

That defines competition. Cooperation needs to become the main focus in the workplace.

If you are a boss and have people that you manage, take a moment to ask yourself a few questions about what type of managerial style you use. Are you the dumb and industrious type? That is, do you not have a clue as to what's going on, but you are telling everybody what to do? Be honest. Or are you the dumb and lazy type, which means you don't have a clue, and don't care about what's going on either?

Are you the smart and industrious type? After dumb and industrious this is the worst one. If you are smart and industrious you will have everyone in your office doing all kinds of busy work and you'll be right in there shouting out orders left and right. The last possibility is smart and lazy. Now, pay attention to this one. The smart and lazy manager kicks back and watches things but does not interfere unless there is a problem. His/ her philosophy is if it's not broke, don't fix it. This way you are not busying yourself to the point that you can't observe what is really going on. Finally, after you have gained some wisdom you can become wise and industrious. In any life situation, but especially in work, you need to know what your hammer is and be able to use it. If you are a boss your hammer is, "You are fired." If you are an employee, it is, "I quit." In a relationship your hammer is "Good bye." You can't use your hammer all the time. You must first elude to the hammer, then show the hammer and if circumstances still don't change use it.

If you are educating yourself then school becomes your job. Like the workplace, creativity and independent thinking are noticeably lacking in this area. The emphasis in education is placed on rote memorization and regurgitation of facts. Humans are unique beings as diverse and varied as the snow flakes which fall from the sky on a cold winter day. Each one of you comes to this planet with your own unique gifts, talents and purpose. The focus of education should then be to stimulate and nurture these unique gifts and talents. This is where the current model of education falls short since the objective has evolved into one of molding young minds to fit into society, rather than having our society be evolved by creative minds. If you look at the curriculum most schools offer today from elementary school to graduate school, the emphasis is placed on making the grade and passing the test. Little attention is paid toward stimulating independent and creative thought, much less encouraging uniqueness or empowering individuals.

By the time most children reach middle school, they are stripped of any individuality they may have possessed when they first began their journey toward self discovery. Children are being strangled by an onslaught of intimidating tests designed to destroy their sense of identity and self confidence. They often struggle to make the grade and please their parents as demonstrated by the popular bumper stickers ("My son/ daughter is an honor student") that parents display on their cars these days. Our educational model focuses on what children are doing wrong rather than what they are doing right! These ever increasing tests and hurdles tell children that society is not interested in what they think, feel or believe, but rather in how they perform under pressure while competing against others. Win at all cost. To some, this unrelenting pressure to succeed is too unbearable as demonstrated by our teenage suicide epidemic.

Recently an eighteen year old girl in our community was hospitalized with nausea, vomiting and severe abdominal pain. For eight days she remained hospitalized perplexing the doctors with her clinical condition. Finally, after multiple diagnostic tests proved non conclusive, I (Elizabeth) was called in to counsel her. Along with a stressful family situation, I learned that this young girl was extremely stressed by the demands of school. Because she had failed to type an English paper, due to her illness, she had received a zero. Since Beth was planning to attend college, this blemish on her student record caused her great emotional dis- ease. As an English teacher myself, I know of the push that exists to prepare seniors for the rigors of college. But why must learning be rigorous? Why does learning have to be competitive and stressful, instead of challenging and fun?

Often children who have been the most obstinate ones emerge as society's greatest artists and contributors because through their rebellion they were able to preserve their unique perspective on life. Why is it that society insists on stripping these incoming souls of the unique gifts and talents they brought with them to help society in the first place? Why is it that we force these young souls to conform to our ineffective social systems rather than letting them lead us into the future? We desperately need individuals with a unique perspective on life to find creative solutions to the devastating problems facing the world today. Monumental issues like crime, violence, disintegration of family values, environmental pollution and terrorism are eating away at our very core. All these are signs that something has gone awry. Societal systems are not doing it right. If these self serving institutions, like education, are failing, what can be done?

Few professions are more important to any society than that of a teacher. Regrettably most teachers today are overworked, underpaid and command very little respect. Their creative ideas are largely ignored by the bureaucrats who make the decisions. Because of these atrocious working conditions, many good teachers have left the profession to the detriment of all. A few exceptional teachers have weathered the unrelenting bureaucratic demands and managed to fan the creative sparkle of their students against all odds. Unfortunately, the greater number of students have lost out and consequently the majority of them find school a boring experience. Imagine! Learning viewed as a boring activity. How can this be? Can you think of anything more exciting than learning about yourself and the world around you? One can only surmise that it must have taken a great deal of effort to dampen the innate curiosity and desire to discover that each soul is born with. The joy of self discovery has been replaced with grade point averages! The satisfaction of self expression and the wonder of unraveling the mysteries of life have been shifted to focusing on competitive test scores, reading levels and social conduct. Schools have all but managed to snuff out the innate burning curiosity and creative sparkle inherent in each soul. I (Elizabeth), remember my first college semester abroad. I traveled to Italy and all at once learning became the most exciting thing in my life. It was no longer confined to the limits of a classroom, books or even the five senses. Knowledge permeated all around me. It abounded in the statutes, architecture and the language spoken by the locals in the streets. As I submersed myself in the culture and history of the country past life memories sprang forth reminding me of other avenues for accessing information. By allowing my own curiosity to lead, I became self motivated and surpassed conventional educational goals. This illustrates how far removed from true learning the typical educational process has become. It seems the piece of paper has gained more significance than the process of attaining it as was so eloquently demonstrated in the movie "Paper Chase."

Not long ago I (Elizabeth) counseled a family who came to me because their child had been diagnosed with an attention deficit disorder and had been put on Ritalin the year prior. The family did not want to put the boy back on Ritalin, but he had been having problems in school. After talking with this thirteen yearold boy it was obvious that he was extremely bright yet, he was failing every subject. When I asked him why he stated, "All we do is copy things, it's so boring." Here was a child that took bicycles apart and put them back together for a hobby and instead of stimulating and challenging his intellect he was taught to copy. Traditional learning based on the current testing system generally employs multiple choice, true or false and fill in the blank type answers. Approximately seventy-five per cent of the material being tested is lost within twenty four hours after taking the test. This means a week after having taken an exam you know as much about the subject as you did before you ever studied for the test. Think of your own life, how much of the material you studied in high school or college can you remember?

This hoop jumping extends to the teachers and other professionals who are required to pass national tests designed to trick recipients rather than weed out those who lack wisdom and good judgement. Some of our most gifted, innovative and natural teachers are prevented from this career because they might have learning disabilities and cannot pass the tests. A friend recounted a story of a woman who was told by the University of Arizona that she should drop out of the education program because she would not be able to pass the tests. She wanted to teach children who had learning disabilities because she suffered from severe dyslexia herself. Can you imagine the impact on a child being taught by this woman? Fortunately, another college in Phoenix did not agree.

In my own situation I (Peter), recall applying to an engineering school in Newark, New Jersey and being told I was not college material because my SAT scores were not high enough. For a while I bought into what I was told and became quite depressed. Fortunately I decided to seek counseling and learned ways to boost my own self esteem eventually following an opportunity to New England where I was accepted by another university. Three years later I graduated as an honor student and was later accepted into a top notch medical school in Boston.

These personal stories illustrate that the current educational methods predominately utilize only left brain activity encompassing only a small portion of your mental capacity. It is no wonder humans typically use less than 6% of their brain power.

Educational models not only do little to encourage using larger portions of the brain, but often discourage it. The time has come to progress to a higher level of education that encompasses the whole individual employing their mental, physical, emotional and spiritual bodies. By using your intuition and going beyond the limits of the intellect, you can tap into the Universal Mind of God and have access to limitless information. This is where the emphasis in education must be placed.

A close look at the curriculum of today's public school systems will easily show private agendas are at play. Did you ever wonder why creativity and independent thought are not given top priority in today's school systems? The multiple choice, true or false and fill in the blanks type questions condition children to respond much the same way as Skinner's pigeons or Pavlov's dogs when given stimuli.

What are your children losing in the process of being educated? What is the nation losing? A society that does not foster creativity and does not promote individual thought is a society easily controlled. This country was founded on well thought principles of true democracy. Preservation of personal freedom was the foundation of the creation of these United States. Children are this nation's most precious resource. If society loses these innately fertile young minds, then surely the future is lost. The Secretary of Labor recently referred to the children of this nation as, "human capital in a global society." Is the education a goal of our country to supply human capital for a global society or is it to help each individual soul in self discovery, unraveling their own unique path and purpose?

It is no secret that private foundations have impactfully influenced the course of education in this country since the early part of this century. Powerful families have made huge amounts of money available to foundations and educational institutions to conduct psychological studies and other research programs. Foundations such as the Rockefeller, Rothschild, Ford, and the Carnegie, to name a few, have used their wealth to influence the direction of education (and other areas) in this country for years. In our current educational system, children are being taught to be followers rather than leaders. Their minds are becoming so conditioned that they are easily manipulated and intimidated by any government.

Many parents across the country have taken steps toward creating home study programs which allow children the unique experience of being taught by someone they love and trust. Home Study has become a vibrant and new force in America. Typically these children do very well in college because their personal interests have guided their education in lieu of conventional systems. Even if you are not a home schooling parent, you need to take responsibility for the education of your children. Encourage your child's interests and talents. If your child shows an interest in music, help him/her to learn to play an instrument. If s/he has an aptitude for science, create an interesting science project and so on.

Budgetary constraints also influence to a large extent what happens in the classroom, thus frequently forcing teachers to teach to the "average" student and leaving little time for individual instruction. But even if more time was available, how creative can teachers be and still complete all the required material? Teachers are trained to use teaching methods developed by institutions whose studies were funded by these powerful foundations previously mentioned. So it becomes a no win situation. To deviate from the norm and use your sense of intuition in teaching would require courage and possible loss of employment as I (Elizabeth), found out when I dared to follow my own methods of teaching.

Currently our educational system operates under the pyramid principle of eliminating candidates until only a select few can make it into the Ivy league schools and become the elite members of society. The rest of the population is often rooted out to serve as the work force for the elite, thus operating from the incorrect age old mentality of slave and master race. What happens to those that make the grade? Do these individuals really have it made?

When I (Peter), was accepted into one of the top medical schools in the nation, I was described by the Dean who addressed our incoming class, as *"la creme de la creme."* He then continued to share some statistical facts that were rather startling: "Most of you will divorce at least once before finishing your training, many of you will become addicted to drugs and/ or alcohol. Those of you who choose surgical specialties will spend more time in a courtroom than most common criminals fighting malpractice lawsuits." Not a cheery life picture. Oh yes, he also said the profession commands high salaries and total dedication. Time, he said, will one day become your worst enemy. By this he meant being a doctor would consume most of my time to the exclusion of other activities.

Medical school training, as with training for other professions, places too much emphasis on how much money the letters behind your name will enable you to earn. What is the point of having money if the other areas of your life are in shambles? Remember, what really counts is evolving all four natures with equal emphasis. As you learn to evolve past emotions then you can take on financial and social evolvement. Too often people believe that amassing a large amount of wealth is all it takes to solve their problems. That's simply not the case. Therefore the emphasis of education should not be placed on obtaining the highest paying job, but rather on learning more about yourself. Once you are on the right path with a solid foundation, everything else will follow with ease, including being of service, as well as financial abundance and the balancing of all four of your natures. Education needs to be an on going activity of self discovery that is constantly challenging the soul, rather than the current model of competition.

Unfortunately, there are those who choose to put their energy toward controlling the masses for the sake of experiencing the rush of power and wealth. This is only an illusion since true power does not come from controlling or manipulating others but from an unwavering connection with the Creator. This inner power comes from the expanded awareness you feel in every cell of your body coming to the realization that you are connected to everything in the manifested Universe.

Educators need to be trained in how to help students find their own power and life purpose through the educational process. They must assist students in making their own choices toward self discovery. New systems need to be established that emphasize creativity and independent thought while nurturing all four natures. A teacher once told me "Wisdom is knowledge used with love and good judgement." This statement symbolizes how valuable educational systems can become once politics is removed from the process of teaching and respect for the young incarnated soul's unique life agenda is emphasized.

Educators need to become facilitators of their students' creative and unique gifts so that everyone can benefit from the contribution these special souls can make to the planet in years to come. It is impossible to talk about education and omit a discussion about creativity. Creativity needs to be the first element in any educational curriculum which unfortunately at present seems to be the last. Creativity is your unique dance with God and your own special way of connecting with the Creator and manifesting Its will here on Earth. As an author of children's books I (Elizabeth), often speak to parents and teachers about empowering children's inner creativity. I tell them that in order to encourage their own child's creativity, they must first empower their own. A parent will not allow their child to experience something they have not allowed themselves to experience. By expanding your own creative abilities you can best serve as an impetus or conduit for your child's creative journey.

What is creativity? Webster defines to create as "to bring something into being." Someone once said "there is no original thought," which agrees with the concept that there is a broader reality that cannot be perceived through the limitations of the five senses but can be tapped into by the use of your imagination. This is the doorway that leads into greater realities. These other realities exist at various levels of consciousness. As you learn to penetrate these levels, your own awareness expands. Many individuals become great creators of songs, poems, drawings, paintings and writings by transcending these levels. They catch a piece of the expanded consciousness and then bring the idea or essence down into the physical realm. These creative works serve as reflections and undeniable proof that greater realities do exist in the cosmos.

It is your willingness to let yourself play in those greater realities that serves as your passport there. Too often playful and imaginative activities are regarded as a waste of time, silly frivolity, when just the opposite is true. You have been taught to believe that productivity is doing something wearisome, boring and that playfulness is a waste of time and not approved of. You must dismiss these notions and change your perspective completely. Is it more valuable to be chasing butterflies in a beautiful meadow than balancing your checkbook? Perhaps one seems to be more enjoyable than the other, but both should be approached with equal respect. A child's work in a sand pile is just as important as an architect building a house.

Playtime is probably the most neglected of all these four activities, usually reserved for children (little people) but seldom enjoyed by adults. As you begin to experience life as a series of opportunities to learn more about yourself, playtime can be identified as an important vehicle through which you can express yourself as a joyful and fun seeking soul on the path of discovering "self." Playing can thus be seen as a way to explore your own Godliness.

Many of you shy away from your own natural inclination to play, feeling that there are more important things to accomplish or others will judge you. Playtime is constantly undermined by the relentless determination to get the job done and move onto the next thing. Playing means a task is left unfinished. Your ego too often succeeds in censoring any desire you may have to be spontaneous and play! Playtime is as important to one's complete spiritual unfoldment as any one other activity, perhaps even more, since it gives the individual the unique opportunity to be spontaneous and creative. This wonderful gift to become a child again leads to feelings of joy, self worth, self love and personal freedom.

Shifting your mind set to playtime, or recreation, immediately gets you out of your head, and into the present moment. You can move beyond the brain's entrapments, expanding past imaginary boundaries and gaining a sense of being one with God. When I (Elizabeth), ride my bike, walk on the beach, or hike a mountain, I become the blades of grass under my feet, the waves that break on the shore, or the boulders that guard my trail. Like the eagle, my consciousness leaves the confines of my physical body and I soar above the world. I become one with all things leaving my thoughts and busyness behind and moving beyond the world of form. Letting yourself play is the first step to this important goal. Most people want to be happy, to feel peaceful and to enjoy their life. But when the urge comes to do something out of the ordinary, the ego steps in and they stop themselves. Imprisoned by social consciousness, they let these precious moments pass by. *Carpe Diem!* "seize the day!" If you cannot allow yourself one moment of happiness, how do you expect to have a whole life full of joy?

Traditionally, many individuals go out on boogie Friday or Saturday night and drink alcohol to unwind and have "fun." Whoever said having fun means drinking alcohol? Those who buy into this belief need a heavy drug such as alcohol to knock out the relentless critical voices which roll around their heads telling them how bad they are or how they don't deserve to enjoy life. Instead, work on your self image and learn to feel worthy to receive an abundance of good things. Playtime is definitely one of those good things.

As I (Elizabeth), am writing these words the sun is setting on the lake which our apartment in Idaho overlooks. Everything is becoming still as the night falls. The ducks are gently gliding across the smooth silvery lake and the mountains cast a blue hue. My soul is soaking in this moment, as I come to the awareness that life is simply a series of moments. At each moment we may choose peacefulness, joy and Oneness with God—or disharmony and unhappiness. The choice is yours. Give yourself the gift of enjoying your life. Take the time to play! Play with your children. Play with your spouse (your playmate). Still yourself enough to hear the voice of the Creator. These are all moments which only you can decide whether or not to seize. *CarpeDiem!*

One of the best models to use in learning how to play comes from nature itself. The dolphin species demonstrates playtime in its purest form. Several years ago while living on Captiva Island, Florida I (Peter), had the privilege to witness these wonderful creatures at play. Every morning I headed for the beach with my writing pad and frequently saw schools of dolphins swimming by, jumping out of the water, performing acrobatics, turning somersaults and simply having a great time. Sometimes I swam close to them and observed their behavior change almost immediately as if wondering whether or not I wanted to join them in their game. Not long ago we visited Mexico and experienced the thrill of swimming, dancing and playing with these magnificent creatures. Unlike homo sapiens, these intelligent, gentle and loving creatures are here on the planet to remind humans how to play.

In the human model the best example of playtime can be seen in observing children, perhaps even your own. Little people, unhindered by big people, can become great teachers in the art of playing. This is especially true with toddlers who have learned the basics of how to move from point A to point B and are still too young to understand what is acceptable social behavior. To these young minds life is nothing more than a huge playground frequently occupied by big people who speak words they do not understand or who sometimes yell alot seldom joining in their world of make believe. Next time the opportunity presents itself, instead of stopping the action, join in and learn something about creativity from your own children.

Ironically, adults tend to get so caught up in their work they often end up mentally, physically, emotionally and spiritually exhausted. At that point all creative energy is blocked by the ego insisting on the expedient completion of a task regardless of how it is done. When this level of saturation is reached, the best solution is to quit whatever you are doing and go play! By playing you allow more creative energy to enter your consciousness, often leading to the solution of a problem previously seen as unsolvable.

I (Peter), treated a patient Susan, a twentythree year old single parent who lived with her two-year old daughter in a small apartment. As soon as I walked into the examining room she began to weep and said "You have to help me. I feel out of control and my daughter is driving me crazy. I want drugs to take these feelings away." I reassured her of my willingness to help find solutions to her problem, but to try other alternatives before using mind altering drugs. She nodded in approval. Her major complaint was that she was angry with her daughter for not obeying house rules and throwing temper tantrums whenever she was disciplined. I asked her "Susan, do you ever play with your daughter?" "Play?" She yelled, "No, she won't listen to me!" During the conversation I suggested that rather than persisting in controlling her daughter's behavior, she could observe her play and join in the fun. I told her that as she was able to develop a life of her own, perhaps she could stop seeing her daughter as a burden and instead learn to enjoy those precious moments together. Children are great teachers in the art of playing. Once you learn how to stop the desire to control them, you are then free to join in the wonder of their creative and imaginative world. The truth is children are here to be your teachers as much as you are to teach them! Learning how to tie your shoes or cross the street is just as important as learning how to build a sand castle or be a fairy princess. If you can allow the power of your children's creative imagination to empower and enrich your life, then both parent and child can win.

Unlike children, the tendency for most big people is to take everything too seriously. Lighten up! Don't take yourself or your relationships or your work so seriously, after all, it's all about self discovery. As you allow yourself to play more you will bring a sense of playfulness to every aspect of your life. Your work will become fun and exciting. A classical example of how this works is how two different surgeons I (Peter), knew operated. During medical school training I spent a summer doing anesthesiology at the Massachusetts General Hospital in Boston and witnessed a famous heart surgeon do several open heart cases per day while listening to music. Throughout the day there seemed to be a sense of cohesiveness in the way personnel in the room related to each other, spear headed by the surgeon's gentle behavior. The work was done very efficiently and yet lightly.

By comparison, I briefly worked in a small hospital some where in the Southwest where the only surgeon in town would insult members of the operating room crew on a regular basis as well as throw temper tantrums whenever something went wrong. This constant verbal abuse created an extremely tense atmosphere to work under and eventually led to a show down between the physician and the hospital administration. When I left the community the hospital was considering his removal from the medical staff because of the many complaints the operating room staff had made. Two different surgeons with different work styles leading to very different results.

Work can be quite enjoyable especially if you are practicing a craft in synchronicity with your life purpose rather than following someone else's footsteps. To achieve this state of mind you must learn to see your work as a great opportunity to express yourself through craftsmanship and playfulness. Just as work can suddenly become a fun activity, depending on your attitude, so can devotional time although here again many individuals may disagree.

Many people take their religion too seriously, believing God does not play. They humble themselves to the Creator with long faces. Do you honestly believe God has no humor? Do you have a sense of humor? Yes? Then it must follow God has humor since you are part of God. Yet, people take their religious beliefs so seriously, often emanating a solemn and pious persona, forgetting devotional time can also be seen as play time with God. Spending time with the Creator in the privacy of your own mind, either in silence or conversation, can be a very enjoyable experience that will surely lighten up your day.

Although fear of God is universally preached, often the end result of this incorrect belief places distance between the you and Creator, when the desired effect is completely the opposite. Can you be close to anyone you fear? As you rejoice by coming to the awareness of your own Godliness, God rejoices also.

THE PATHWAY HOME

The Godliness of playing can be seen in toddlers whose minds have yet to be tainted with social concepts such as fear of God, fear of Hell and so on. To them life is joy. If you haven't already noticed, their warm innocent smiles are highly contagious which frequently results in the tearing down the emotionless mask of social consciousness that many big people wear when talking to God. You must become as a little child to enter the kingdom of heaven. As an evolving soul one of your jobs is to see and experience the world as a child full of wisdom and self love. This is a task that few individuals ever master except those who call themselves eternal children. These people are able to keep a sense of playfulness and joy as they go through life's lessons mostly focusing on the best of a situation rather than the worst. In other words, they see the glass half full rather than half empty.

In the Western World devotion is probably the least thought of activity. By contrast, in the East devotion is a common part of everyday life. In the Middle East for example, five times daily, Moslems prostrate themselves towards the East in prayer. Cries of praise for Allah ring out across the land. In the far East, Monks and peasants alike sit in quiet meditation, taking time out from their daily routine to be with God. In the Western World we are too busy running around to take time out to be with God. Devotion is your way of connecting with and speaking to God. A sincere act of devotion immediately puts you in a state of bliss. It is through devotion that you are reminded that all things are interconnected and you are part of God. Through the very holy act of devotion you see God in all things: the dishes you wipe dry, the sun as it sets, your child's face as you wipe a tear from his/her eye.

Unfortunately, devotion tends to take on the sense of a duty like catechism. In truth it is a gift you give to yourself. The gift of spending time with the Creator. Meditation and prayer are ways to connect with God. In meditation it is best if you choose a certain time of the day, for example, early morning. As soon as you rise, get yourself into a comfortable position and begin your meditation. Focusing on a mantra will help to still the mind and bring it into focus. The mantra we use is SAT NAM, which means: Truth be Its name. Bring your focus to your third eye, the space between your physical eyes in the center of your forehead and repeat the words SAT NAM as you exhale. Ideally, you should tithe ten percent of your time in devotional activities. That is approximately two and half hours a day. You needn't spend all your devotional time in meditation. Any activity can be made into a devotional one, as you evolve you will realize that your whole life is spent in endless devotion. Your life will become an on going love affair between you and the Creator. The joy of being of service and being connected to all things will fill you.

The easiest way to start getting a sense of devotion is to take a walk in an area filled with nature. I (Elizabeth), usually enjoy a stroll at sunset. I watch all the creatures around me preparing for nightfall and gaze at the sun as it softly slips from the sky, casting beautiful colors around me. I feel connected with all living things: the birds, the trees, the grass. Prayer is also an excellent form of devotion as it immediately softens you and puts you into a receptive mode.

Guidance and comfort are always within your reach. Begin to develop your own relationship with God.

Use your own words when you speak with God. Get to know God, inside and out. Prayers can be beseeching, affirming—anything you want. Talk to God as often as you can. Give thanks for being alive, for the air you breath, the sun that shines, for the smallest of things. Being grateful is a most uplifting activity. Feel God around you and within you. Throughout the day constantly keep your focus on God. The more time you spend being with God, the more you will come to know God. Another powerful aspect of devotion is its ability to soften you enough to receive grace. Grace descends from the heavens. In order to receive grace from God you need only humble yourself. Anyone who can humble themselves is worthy to receive this outpouring of grace from the Creator. Grace is a marvelous aspect of God. It is that for giving, nurturing and empowering energy that can catapult you quantum leaps along your spiritual path. Grace is given, not asked for!

When I (Elizabeth), think of devotion, I can't help but think of our Native American brothers and sisters who spent much of their time in devotional practices. They respected and nurtured the Earth and her spirits. Much of their devotion was and still is expressed through song and dance. I recall performing a liturgical dance with my cousin in a church in Italy. As I danced "spirit" moved through me. It was a beautiful act of devotion. Be free and creative in the way you express your devotion. You may choose to express it through song, dance, a work of art, or loving silence. Try and find a sense of devotion in everything you do, even the most mundane of activities. For example, cleaning the house can be elevated to a level of spiritual heights by performing it with devotion.

As you evolve you will bring the healing power of devotion into every aspect of your life. You will perform your work with devotion, make love with devotion, every moment of your life will be an opportunity to further know God through endless acts of loving devotion. By merging devotion with self responsibly in every area of your life, you will increase your awareness and move with ease down the pathway Home.

Section Six:

The Pathway Home

*The job is easy Do what's in front of you
be still and know . . You are God.*

CHAPTER 13
SELF RESPONSIBILITY AND DOORS

It should be clear by now that one of the themes throughout this book is becoming whole through self responsibility. Regardless of the specific nature or activity being discussed, self responsibility is a crucial step in obtaining freedom and expanded awareness. By following the foundation laid out for you in this book and by evolving and balancing all four of your natures, you can escape the entrapments of society and move into the light of spiritual freedom.

To evolve your four natures you must assume responsibility for each nature. In matters of physical wellness, if you live a life of excess without regard for your physical temple you must deal with the consequences of your irresponsible actions. Becoming aware of what your body needs to maintain balance and optimum health is your responsibility. In regards to emotional wellness, realizing you are responsible for how you feel and choosing to extract yourself from the emotional roller coaster ride of life by focusing internally rather than externally, is a starting point. By choosing to remain in a constant state of peacefulness you will find equanimity in all things, freeing yourself. Mental wellness is achieved when you are able to observe your actions and regard situations of emotional imbalance as lessons presented to you to demonstrate where you are losing contact with the Creator. You will then be able to identify behavioral patterns "borrowed" from parents, teachers, religions and society at large and move beyond them into the one point focus of Godrealization. In spiritual matters placing your trust in so called spiritual leaders from the ranks of organized religion has resulted in putting more distance between you and the Creator. For centuries billions of souls have come to believe they must go through other individuals who identify themselves as servants of the Lord in order to receive grace from God. You must take on the responsibility of forging your own relationship with God and determining what spirituality means to you. Countless labyrinths have developed in modern society whose focus is to render the individual powerless and interfere with his/her self discovery and pursuit of happiness. It is your responsibility to see behind the mask of illusion the government and social systems project and become independent of these decaying institutions. In short, it all amounts to: Always being selfresponsible in all areas of the human condition is the surest way to become fully realized individuals!

A patient I (Peter), saw recently is a good example of the dis- ease humans take on when they fail to assume the responsibility of addressing all four of their natures. She was a thirty two year old, who had seen numerous doctors over the past three years for a painful vaginal condition. According to her own verbal history, "They tried everything on me." I asked her if she was sexually active to which she responded in a loud voice, "No, I'm Not!" I continued, "When was the last time you had intercourse?" She gave the precise date of March 24th, 1989, when she began to have symptoms. So I continued, "Would you tell me what happened then?" She became quite nervous and agitated then said, "What is this? Why do you want to know?" I told her, "Do you think there might be a connection between whatever happened to that relationship and your symptoms now?" She blurted out, "That son of a bitch was sleeping with another woman!" We went on for a while to discuss those feelings, and how they related to her symptoms. In the end she said, "Thank you for doing the mental thing, but I still have something wrong, can't you see?" She was right. She did have something physically wrong: an incredibly tender, reddened vaginal opening caused by the tremendous emotional trauma of ending a relationship that was very important to her. This patient demonstrates what can happen when one tries to compartmentalize the human condition and look to someone else, in this case a doctor, to take the pain away. Believing you can ignore the physical signs and emotions your body gives forth, is the quickest way to become dis- eased.

Regrettably many members of the medical profession will not even attempt to make a mind bodydis- ease connection and simply proceed to treat the last step in a long chain of events instead of exploring the whole person. Healers must first take responsibility for looking at their own lives and attending to what needs to be healed, then they must address all aspects of the patient, instead of acting as technophysicians—mechanics of the human body. The current trend in treating an "emotional" patient is to refer him/her to another technospecialist who will categorize the emotional disturbance according to a manual which contains hundreds of categories for mental illnesses. From that day on, that individual is stuck with a diagnosis, a label, which s/he will carry for life. Why?

It is the responsibility of healers to stop perpetuating the myth that body, mind and spirit are separate. Healers, physicians, therapists etc. must look at the whole patient regardless of their specialty or particular area of interest. Diet and nutrition are as important to a psychotherapist as emotional wellness should be to an internist. Many mental health care professionals criticize physicians for not dealing with patient's emotions, while they ignore vital areas such as how the patient's diet affects the patient's mood swings.

The public is told that modern medical science knows much more about healing today than it did 3,000 years ago. If the highest definition of true healing is to help spirit flow more freely through the physical body, is modern medicine accomplishing this goal? Healers must cease practicing with blinders, focusing on one organ, emotion, belief, or spiritual philosophy and treat the whole patient coming from a place of integrating spirit into the physical body.

This does not mean the healer cannot provide temporary relief through the use of drugs, surgery or any means which is compatible with the patient's belief systems. But if deeper changes do not occur, the dis- ease will return. Both patients and healers must assume the responsibility of going beyond the current healthcare model.

If a patient comes to me (Peter), with a physical problem, I use all my skill and knowledge to assist her in healing herself. I also know there is a reason for her illness. My job is to help her recognize the patterns which brought about her illness, and if necessary remove the dis- eased tissue surgically. The patient's responsibility is to participate in all major decisions regarding her own health recovery plan. A wide variety of information needs to be presented so they can know their options and make intelligent decisions.

If you become ill, you are responsible for looking at yourself, your lifestyle, your emotional imbalance, and your physical actions to see what is causing your illness. If you are a two pack a day smoker and one day you begin to cough up blood, is it someone else's responsibility that you now have lung cancer? If you allow others to treat you with harshness and internalize your emotions until it develops into an acute abdominal bleeding ulcer, are they responsible or are you responsible for the outcome? If you were physically, emotionally and mentally abused by a parent, does it give you the right to abuse your children? If you disconnect yourself from the love of the Creator, is it God's fault? Self responsibility begins with a conscious recognition that particular patterns are not working for the individual. This brings about the option to choose something different; a conscious choice to change.

There is a reason for every illness you create for yourself. Even the common cold gives type A people viable permission to take a rest from the world that they may otherwise not permit themselves to take. An illness can often be identified as serving some purpose to the afflicted. It gives you permission to rest, to reflect and to receive nurturing from others. You can therefore demand attention from other individuals as well as love, support and emotional nourishment. As you also saw in the chapter on "Greed" it can bring about monetary income from lawsuits. Other social systems that support a dis- eased state include social security, workmen's compensation and sick leave, just to name a few. These social systems often support illness and irresponsibility. This unfortunate set of circumstances is the result of healthcare systems which absolve the patient from any responsibility regarding their own health.

What about wellness? Is there anything to be gained by prevention? Do you really think that you were meant to be sick, to suffer physical pain? The natural state of the body is perfect health. So, why do many individuals choose to suffer? Is it to pay for their perceived inadequacies? Are you somehow punishing yourself for your "sins"? Can you give up the notion you are bad and believe you are worthy to receive an abundance of good things? Becoming whole and feeling healthy is part of these good things.

Sin, incorrect thinking, is a misperception an individual has about himself/

herself and/or others. Incorrect thinking creates negative energy patterns which manifests in the world as negative matter. This matter is physically seen as dis- ease, poverty, anger, confusion, jealousy, defensiveness, apathy and unhappiness. Sin takes you down a path contrary to the very nature you represent: The image of God. It is your responsibility to infuse every area of your life with correct thinking.

Your true nature is to be happy, joyful, excited, beautiful, compassionate, childlike and wise. Have you ever felt like that before? Ever had a glimmer of your true nature? I (Peter), have. In fact, I feel that way a lot. You might ask how did I do it? What changed my life? It was a choice I made. You may ask how can I feel that way when the world is crumbling around me? How can I permit myself to feel joy with all the human suffering? I can because to reflect on human suffering would only perpetuate the illusion that we are powerless and separate from God. Why support the belief that happiness and health are outside us? Why not accept the truth that God is in each and every one of us, and that the nature of God is in every cell of our bodies. Acknowledge the "perfect reflection" of God existing within you. You are responsible for seeking out this truth.

As a medical student I (Peter), was bombarded with facts relating to the pathophysiological aspects of dis- ease, very little emphasis was placed on preventive medicine and how nutrition plays a key role in maintaining physical wellness. You are what you eat, drink, breathe and think and therefore responsible for what you put into your body and mind. Relaying nutritional information helps patients prevent dis- ease and develop a life long pattern of responsible eating habits. In this manner healers can help patients to make responsible choices.

Do you believe you can live to be 150 or 200 years old or more? I believe it is possible. The Bible tells many stories of individual's lives lasting over 500 years. How did they accomplish what appears to most individuals as an impossible feat? The answer lies in their direct relationship to God and the spaceship called Earth. Mother Earth is to some individuals their dearest, maternal or feminine force that provides everything they need for nourishment. Think about it: everything you have comes from Mother Earth in one form or another. The food you eat, the clothes you wear, the car you drive. The attitude and spiritual respect for this home has changed in the minds of many individuals during recent times. Reverence for the life sustenance that is provided from our living home is all but forgotten. This incorrect perception has cut the longevity out of our own lives. The current attitudes and perceptions are reflected in all aspects of modern day living: people eat to fill the void within themselves rather than eating to nurture their bodies. This misperception of food, seen not as nourishment but rather physical pleasure, is reflected in an overweight society immersed in dieting. People refuse to see the connection food and daily habits have on their emotions and physical body. Along with the nutritional value of food we need to be aware of the ingredients they contain. Additives, poisons, preservatives, pesticides, hormones and the very water which is added to their content, adds to their nutritional value. Carcinogenic substances added to many food products and drinking water are taken into your body. You must become responsible for the food you eat by simply saying no to products which are harmful to your temple. We must also become responsible for our environment. What are these pesticides doing to our streams and rivers, and to our land? How is greed effecting our environment? What is happening to our forests, oceans, and soil? If we cannot sustain our planet how will our planet sustain us? Like the cancer cell killing the host, our irresponsible behavior is destroying that which feeds and nurtures us.

The pattern of irresponsibility begins even before childhood. It begins with the parent's decision to become parents. So often individuals simply procreate without giving much thought as to the awesome responsibility they are assuming by bringing a child into the world. Many people have children simply because "it's the thing to do." You get married and have children. Perhaps your parents or religion encourages this behavior. I see young folks nineteen years old, and younger getting pregnant without a clue as to the responsibility involved. The result is a society that is not responsibly raising their young. Teachers, schools systems and social programs are over worked because they are assuming this responsibility. Little people are not getting their mental, emotional, spiritual, and in many cases, physical needs met. We are literally killing our children. While visiting Louisville, Kentucky this past summer, I (Elizabeth), was told by my parents about a five month old baby who had been given to her father to drop off at day care. He forgot all about her, never dropping her off or even taking her out of the car when they arrived at his workplace. He even went out to lunch with a friend and returned to his job with the baby still strapped into the back seat. Because of the sweltering heat and humidity, the baby died. The man was acquitted because in everyones heart they knew that they themselves could make the same mistake. The sign of this event and countless other events similar to this one which plague our headlines daily, is that we are neglecting our children. If their physical needs are not being met, what about their emotional, mental and spiritual needs? Our children are the future. If you are thinking about having children do so only because you truly want to, not to make your parents, grandparents, or because all your friends are having babies, or to create a larger congregation for your church. It's a tough job. It is difficult to meet the needs of your four natures and those of your children. Give yourself time to learn and grow, to evolve yourself before you take on responsibility for other souls.

Parents who are responsible are the best living examples for teaching self responsibility to their children. Children need to be empowered to make choices and learn from the consequences of their actions. Parents can then help children to make wiser choices the next time round. Think of how much more evolved our society would be if people were held accountable for their choices at an early age.

For every action an individual takes, there is an equal or opposite reaction. This is the Law of Karma. Whether you are aware of it or not, nothing happens to you by accident. The very conditions of your present life's situations are the results of your thoughts and actions of the past manifested in the present. With this understanding the act of revenge, or making yourself responsible for teaching someone else a lesson becomes redundant. Everyone will receive just repayment for their actions. Therefore you need not concern yourself by avenging someone who has wronged you. To take responsibility for something that is not yours similarly creates karma. Look after yourself and let others look after themselves.

Beyond self responsibility comes the area of social responsibility. Within the realm of social responsibility you find the single most powerful tool, or weapon, which exists in modern society: television. Practically every household in the U.S. and now in many parts of the world have at least one television. It has become more than just a simple pastime reaching the status of an addiction in many households. People indiscriminately tune in while they are working, exercising or eating. Some individuals go as far as to turn the television on just because they can't stand to be alone. The minute you sit in front of what is affectionately called the "boob tube", you enter a passive state of hypnosis. Television relaxes the mind so that it becomes amenable to suggestions. This explains why people can sing the jingles to most every popular advertisement seen on the media. Advertising has obviously been a great success otherwise corporations wouldn't spend billions of dollars each year thinking up new ways to get you to buy their products. I (Elizabeth), remember the famous scene from the movie "Network" where a prophetic newscaster tells his audience that they dress like the tube, think like the tube, even raise their families like the tube. He explains to his captive audience that the tube isn't reality, it is just an illusion, perhaps the greatest illusion of all. Then he instructs everyone to turn off their televisions.

Take a moment to loosen the grip television has on you and your family's life by turning it off for a few days and observe if you or any of your family members go through a withdrawal period. Observe the products you buy, your political beliefs and opinions of world events. Television is undoubtedly the most powerful tool that exists in modern society to mold public opinion. Nowadays, public opinion is where the power lies. If you manage to have public opinion on your side, the battle is won. Look to history to review this truism.

It is amazing even today how many people are intimidated by public opinion and are afraid of being "politically incorrect." To be self responsible means you do not become someone else's pawn. You must have the courage to follow your own sense of what is right, even if it may not be the popular choice. You must also be responsible for what you allow to enter your mind, and not allow yourself to be conditioned. You must learn to employ "the correct use of will" and have the courage not to surrender your will to others. While it is important to have a cursory knowledge of world affairs, use your sense of intuition to determine whether a piece of information is indeed the truth. Do not be fooled by any political leader or become embroiled in someone else's agenda. Strive to see the truth in all things.

It is important for those who have the power of the media behind them to use it responsibly. Imagine all that is happening on our planet and yet all the newscasters focus on the same thing: politics, murders, disasters and war. This bias in reporting reinforces the misperception that we live in a dangerous world and you need someone (the government) to take care of you. This way the illusion of fear is perpetuated. Fearful people are easily controlled. You must not let a few reporters and newscasters serve as your eyes and ears. You must choose programs that are insightful and informative and use your intuition to decipher the truth. You must seek the truth for yourself from within.

The movie industry still largely functions dependent of politics. Throughout this book we have cited several movies as examples of how information is leaked to the public. Many screenwriters and directors are blessed with enough intuition in their storytelling to expose much of the secret workings of the government. Censorship is being widely sought to eliminate our last link to any bearance of truth. The highest purpose of a film, as with any art form, is to transform the soul. Film should inform, educate, entertain, illuminate and evolve your audience. Through the phenomenon of synchronicity information is being disseminated to the masses through movies. Unfortunately, there are individuals within the industry who abuse this powerful medium and use it only to further their own financial status, propagandize, and/or further enslave audiences in ignorance. It is interesting how a movie like "Outbreak" was released just a few weeks before the Ebola virus appeared in Africa. In the movie, Dustin Hoffman's character repeatedly leaks out the military's use of viruses as powerful weapons. Movies like "Roswell" and "Intruders" expose the government's involvement in a major cover up of aliens. "The Philadelphia Experiment" tells of the government tampering with time travel and its deadly consequences. The government's highly evolved progress in human cloning is revealed in movies such as "Anna to the Infinite Power" and "The Boys from Brazil." Fiction or fact?

Are you beginning to assume responsibility for your life? Are you beginning to wake up? As you move away from old patterns of incorrect thinking towards the freedome of correct thinking many new awareness and opportunities will arise. You must become aware of the signs and doors that point you further along your pathway toward spiritual unfoldment. As the seeker of spiritual enlightenment awakens, s/he begins to realize that there is a certain rhythm by which all things, large and small, are played out in the Universe. What does it mean to be in rhythm with the Universe? You are all part of a cosmic orchestra expressing yourself with your own unique tone. You must first learn your tone well enough so that you may harmonize it with the rest of the Universe.

The first step in this process of increased awareness is to realize that the Universe is feminine in nature and therefore hidden. It speaks to you through symbols. Just like the markings on this paper are symbols which you have learned to interpret, so must you learn to decipher the way the Universe communicates. It is quite simple. The problem arises when your brain gets in the way intellectualizing rather than intuiting the information being presented to you. The Universe speaks to you in very simple ways: through bumper stickers, Tshirt, license plates, and out of the mouths of those around you. The next time someone comes to your door, or is talking to you, listen to the higher meaning of what they are saying. If someone from a religious group comes to your door offering to show you the way out of hell and into the arms of Jesus, they are just reminding you to stay plugged in. When we were in Arizona we were told to move to Idaho, every other person we met was from Idaho. Every car on the road had an Idaho license plate. We often hiked the Superstition Mountains outside Phoenix and found ourselves turning off the freeway onto Idaho Road. Just as your dreams are symbolic, so too is your waking state. In fact, everything you do is a reflection of the greater reality of spirit. Search out the highest meaning in all things. When you learn to correctly interpret Universal signs these doors present opportunities for growth. You need to move through the doors that open along your path. Similarly, if a door is closing move away from it. You can be sure another door will open for you somewhere else.

As you learn the process of surrendering yourself to God, you come to the awareness that each of you represents a minuscule component, a cell, within a cosmic organism that is part of the Creator. Life experiences are presented to you for the purpose of expanding your awareness and thus coming one step closer to God. As you rise above the limits of your own brain and ego, your consciousness will begin to blend with the Creator's giving you moments of peak experience and expanded awareness.

Some of you may immediately question the idea of surrendering yourself to God as contradicting the concept of a free will. Everyone has free will. The correct use of will comes from correct thinking. Most people give away their will at the wrong moment or use it incorrectly as willful children. If you are on your way to exercise and someone stops you to chat and you stay and talk even though you're late, you have just given up your will. Although this seems to be a minor incident, it and others like it multiplied hundreds of times in your daily life adds up to you being diverted from your spiritual path through the lack of the correct use of will. As you evolve you will learn that when you surrender your will to God, you will always be moved in the direction of your soul's highest spiritual purpose. In other words, management will never steer you wrong! For those who in this time frame are willing to keep their original covenant (agreement) made with the Creator approximately six thousand years ago to follow God's Will, they shall reap the rewards. For those who choose to do that now, they shall have dominion over the Earth and life everlasting.

The problem lies in the way society has evolved, placing all the emphasis on materialistic accomplishments, totally forgetting to allow the individual enough room to ask the question, is this life experience in the best interest of my soul's growth?

Somehow most Western societies have come to accept the false premise that the spiritual world is separate from the physical world. Many so called "spiritual" individuals make the mistake of excluding spirituality from their daily activities. Their spirituality remains confined to the realms of lofty ideals and they fail to bring these spiritual principles into their bodies and their everyday lives, effecting solid and concrete changes. Remember everything is spiritual. "It is all One".

To best illustrate the concept of cosmic doors, I (Peter), will share two personal incidents where the first case demonstrates my own ego superseding a Higher Will and the second demonstrates what happens when you surrender to God. Several years ago we decided our house in Central Florida was not big enough for the two of us. Our friends and family members loved the house because it sat on a great big lake and was quite comfortable to live in. In the opinion of most individuals who saw it, the house was perfect and fun to be in. One of the features it had was a boat ramp which we often used to enjoy various water activities. To us, however, the house was missing something which at that point in our lives we both felt we needed. This missing component was space and more land to build the house of our dreams.

We started looking for land and found what we thought was the ideal spot to build our dream home. A friend of ours who used to be a realtor served as our negotiator and soon it became apparent the deal was not flowing. We felt the asking price was too high and the property did not include access to a beautiful river, which flowed nearby. Back and forth we went until finally after many weeks of negotiating we agreed on a price which included an easement to the river. The property was heavily wooded with gorgeous elm and oak trees, some of which needed to be cleared in order to make space for the house. We hired an interesting old man who did the landscaping and was considered by many an artist when it came to creating a living space that was in harmony with nature. Within a few short weeks this man and I (Peter), became friends. One night while visiting his home we sat out side watching the beautiful Florida skyline. He said to me, "Peter, if I were you I would not spend so much money building this house right now. We're in the middle of a recession and, in my opinion, the best thing for you to do is to hold on to your money and stay where you are." This kind soul, who a few months later died of lung cancer (he was a heavy smoker), had warned me and yet I still was not listening.

Meanwhile, my wife while studying to obtain a real estate license, mentioned to her instructor the property we had purchased. He said to her "Sell the lot and whatever you do, don't build a house now." Again another warning given to us by the Universe through her instructor which we did not heed. During this same time period we received several other clues not to build the house, however, our attachment to the idea of a "dream home" was so strong we chose to ignore all signs and went on to construct it. During construction we experienced several major setbacks which ultimately lead to a dispute between ourselves and the builder dealing with cost overruns. Finally, thirteen months later, the house was finished thirty thousand dollars over budget. The first night in the house we discovered a gas leak that nearly blew the place up. The next day we noticed the drinking water had a terrible smell. This new problem had developed since the water was tested by the man who dug the well. Four thousand dollars later, after purchasing new components for the water purification system, we ended up with decent water to drink.

Approximately eighteen months later, the course of our lives took a dramatic turn which meant we had to sell a highpriced home in a depressed real estate market. My old friend had warned me three years earlier but my ego said no. We paid the karmic consequences of our decision to go against the flow of things. It took over two years to sell "our dream house" at a price much below what it had been appraised for or even cost to build. When a door is not opening for you, the best thing to do is to walk away. By refusing to flow with the Creator's Will, I ended up paying dearly with a great many moments of unhappiness, despair and financial loss when I could have instead chosen an easier path and remained in the lake house which we truly enjoyed and had sold for a nice profit.

By comparison, I want to share with you another example which took place two years later in New Mexico. By this time my awareness of a greater reality and the concept of cosmic doors was much more a part of my daily living and so the out come was quite different. I don't have to tell those of you who have visited the mountains in northern New Mexico how beautiful they are. While living in Santa Fe my wife and I discovered a little town called Jemez Springs that honestly looked so pretty it belonged on the list of the ten most beautiful spots in the Rocky Mountains. We found a small but cute cabin for sale that an attorney used on week ends. It needed some work. The cabin was very private and had a nice feel to it. We looked at each other and we knew immediately we were supposed to live there.

That same weekend we signed a contract and thirty days later the cabin was ours. First, we had to upgrade it since it had only been used as a weekend home and so we hired various people to remodel the bathroom, install new carpet, appliances and a new heating system. Three months later the cabin was finished and it looked beautiful. The cabin was well within our means so we actually saved money while enjoying the many trails, various hot springs, and the historic bath house in the village down the mountain. At night we watched the stars that crowded the heavens and cozied up in front of our fireplace. It is difficult to imagine another placed I loved so much as that 1,200 sq. ft. cabin, confirming the old saying that life is most beautiful when it's kept simple.

Just about the time we were starting to feel real comfy, new signs began to appear which heralded our departure from New Mexico. At first we both ignored thesigns, but as signs do, they kept on coming, until one day a wake up call to both of us finally arrived. Our septic system was clogged up with roots that had grown into the main pipe. Suddenly our little heaven on Earth became an anchor trying to keep us from evolving our souls and proceeding on to the next assignment. We still resisted the signs and again tried to ignore them but to no avail. The washing machine broke next then the swamp cooler and so on until we were convinced by management that it was time to move on. So very reluctantly, we put the cabin up forsale at a price we were certain we would not get anytime soon. Four weeks later a couple agreed on the asking price and the cabin was sold.

Another important sign which manifested around this time was the sale of a condominium we purchased in Santa Fe when we first moved West. After deciding to move to Albuquerque we seized the opportunity to rent out the unit in a market where housing is at a great shortage. Our real estate investment paid off and we were able to rent the condo for twice the monthly mortgage payment. Precisely at the same time we put the cabin up for sale the condo lessee decided to move out. Immediately we recognized the sign and put this unit up for sale as well. Four weeks later the condominium sold for the asking price. Judging from the results, our interpretation of the signs was right although part of us was still resisting the change. The cosmic doors, symbolized by ordinary life events, had remained open for us to go through them with ease. Timing is every thing! So as long as your timing is not too far off, the door(s) will remain open and it will be easy to identify the path of least resistance.

The ability to let go and become totally detached from the physical world is one of the prerequisites to reaching Godrealization. To have the courage to say no to your intellect and overcome your fear of the unknown is also of paramount importance in reaching this goal. You must trust God enough to follow the path wherever it takes you and know all along you are being taken care of. Regardless of the specific situation which may arise along your path, such as a change of life partners, change of careers, change of lifestyle, change of address and so on, the importance lies in your ability to "see" the doors as they are presented to you and act upon them in a timely fashion. This leads us to a key question: what if you lack suffcient awareness to "see" the door that appears along your path? Do you get another chance? The answer is a resounding yes! God has infinite patience. The time-space illusion that you are part of, exists only in this three dimensional world. So stop beating yourself up for something you may have missed in the past and focus on the now. It does not take much time to figure out society does not work in harmony with these universal principles. It matters not what society believes, it only matters what you believe. Are you ready to consciously become part of the Great Plan? Are you prepared to perform God's Will? Are you brave enough to trust that everything in the manifested world is really an illusion of a greater reality, which works symbolically for you so that you can learn more about yourself? Are you humble enough to bow your will to that of the Creator's? The Great Plan includes your spiritual evolvement because as you evolve, representing the microcosm, the Creator also evolves representing the macrocosm. As above, so below. The rule is simple: do what's in front of you! Regardless of the activity your job is to flow with the Universal current, wherever it takes you. This can be a frightening experience if you are one of those individuals who is always needing to be in control. The truth is you are not in control of anything. You can only place your trust in the Creator and move forward. Nothing in the manifested Universe remains the same. There is no such thing as status quo, therefore, if you are not moving forward you are dying backwards! How often have you found yourself "stuck" in a certain situation because of your unwillingness to let go when you had a chance to do so? I (Peter), certainly have, many times, in fact I have given you some examples already. After all this time of doing what I was taught, i.e., if at first you don't succeed, try, try again, I learned there is another much easier way. If you don't succeed, let it go! If after some time has passed and you still feel the urge, try again. If it is still not flowing, forget about it and go on to something else. Always take the path of least resistance in everything you do!

Another rule to look at when deciding whether you should continue to follow a certain path is to look at the results of that specific activity. If the activity you are doing is allowing you the opportunity to learn more about yourself, then by all means continue until there is nothing else to learn from it. This rule is most difficult to follow when it comes to relationships. As we have already discussed in another chapter, in this area many individuals seem to over extend their stay and consequently get stuck in certain patterns that perpetuate conflict between the two partners. Fear of abandonment is what keeps many individuals unable to evolve the current relationship they are in or even in some case to move on to another partnership.

The same rules mentioned earlier also apply to relationships where the individual should take the path of least resistance. Keep it simple and do what's in front of you. Use your intuition as much as possible and when in doubt do as little as possible. If the relationship is not nurturing your four natures as you and your partner continue the process of self discovery, then you should ask management whether or not you should remain in partnership. Often the answer, expressed through symbols, will come to your consciousness. At that point the decision is yours and yours alone. Will you continue to follow the lower aspects of your will, plagued by worn out belief systems and external cues which come from a society disconnected from God, or will you follow the Divine Will which is the unalterable will sent down from the Creator? By following the latter, the pathway Home is inevitable.

CHAPTER 14

HOME

As you begin to follow God's Will and others do the same, humankind will enter an exciting and unique future. Global transmutation of consciousness will be aided by 144,000 souls who will transgress the levels and disseminate information as fully committed Light workers. Let us shift into the future and see what a world of Universal citizens living in harmony with the Creator's Will would be like as their actions come from a place of self responsibility, wholeness and inner peace.

The highest spiritual symbol of the beehive is the symbol of the Masters. Bees work together harmoniously. Each bee in the colony has at least one job to do, sometimes more as in the female bees or worker bees. These bees do everything from nursing the young and house keeping, to construction, ventilating, guarding of the hive and cross pollination. Bees work together efficiently and cooperatively, humming along as they busily carry out their duties with devotion and loyalty. While performing their service to their hive, they also do a greater service to our planet by cross pollinating flowers and other plant life. All the collaborative efforts of the bees culminate in the production of a golden nectar honey.

What if we as humans could learn from these small creatures how to live and work in complete cooperation, devotion, and harmony with the Creator? What if we could learn to work together, where everyone has a job that results in the production of a golden nectar—The Creator's Divine Will? Some critics would say the human condition is much too difficult to overcome and Home is a fairy tale unobtainable or perhaps only reachable by saints and gurus but not you. The daily jolts of modern society do not allow for the individual in today's world to reach this state of bliss. This simply is not true.

We are reaching an extraordinary time in the history of our planet when the energies are such that who so ever chooses to evolve need only reach their hand out to God. By following a path of correct thinking and correct action, you will evolve mentally, physically, emotionally, spiritually, as well as financially and socially, and reach this goal. By choosing to evolve, sloughing off the limitations of past belief systems, you allow more Light to enter your body. This increased energy in the form of Light radiation will then boost your body and allow it to reach new levels of spiritual awareness never before possible.

There are many who will not choose to go with this flow but instead resist this powerful energy. In our journeys around the planet we have observed certain vortices or areas where spiritual energies are exceptionally strong. In these areas you find an assortment of souls who have been drawn to them and the different ways they react to these energies. Some people suck up the energy and simply bask in the light but never transfer it into some useful concrete activity to benefit themselves or others. Others draw in the energy and use it, translating it into some tangible means of serving our planet. The third category are the people drawn to these areas but don't know what to do with these energies. Instead of releasing their personal limitations and evolving their physical vehicles to let in more of the Light, they instead choose to block it. These people are usually heavy drinkers and/or drug users.

As you learn to move beyond form (the physical body), you will become more sensitive to the energies around you. People will become known to you by their energy rather than the "garbs of their ego." You will be able to sense energy patterns in places you visit (in the physical and non physical) and learn to discern and blend with these energies. When you enter a place either in nature or in society, become aware of the vibration at which the area resonates. Is it a high vibration or is it low? Is the energy comfy and cozy or does it pack power? Is it harmonious or disintegrative? Become aware of the energy radiating from our Sun. Does it move in waves? Is it stronger or more intense at certain times than others?

As you grow closer to your goal of Home you will more easily move beyond form and be able to see the true essence of all things. You will realize the interconnectedness of all things in a manner never before comprehended and come to know form as only a manifestation of spirit. When you can resonate from this high place then you can come together with your brothers and sisters on this planet, soul to soul, rather than personality to personality. You will not be preoccupied with being too fat, having a bad hair day, or other trivial matters. These thoughts will dissolve into a greater awareness that you are much more than your physical form. You will go beyond form to a place of spirit. The key to this level of awareness is to learn how to control the brain. It is your brain that keeps you locked into form. That is why it is helpful to meditate and use a mantra, or go for walks in nature.

Intellectuals among you may find it extremely difficult to accept that the human can go beyond the physical boundaries of his/her brain. To understand the greater mysteries of the Universe you must leave the brain behind. To fully comprehend the concept of time you must lose the brain and any preconceived ideas you learned about time being linear. Those of you who can humble yourselves and tap into the Universal Mind will come to learn how time really works.

In your quest for evolvement you may find that many of your friends, family members and even your partner will not understand you. Out of fear, they may try to hold you back. Let yourself become detached from any situations or people that are not spiritually uplifting. Give yourself space, physical as well as mental and emotional space, and time to create new patterns of behavior. Some of these people may fall along the wayside, along with activities you no longer enjoy. Not to worry. You are not losing sight of life's pleasures but are instead moving toward a greater awareness of the inward joy life brings. Even if you find yourself alone, remember you are never alone, but All One. Eventually you may have a relationship with these individuals free from social expectations and based on unconditional love and acceptance. Remember to allow each soul their own pace of self unfoldment. This does not mean that if your partner is not unfolding at the same speed you are that the relationship is over. Give each other time and space. Be accepting of the other while pursuing your own life path. Don't be afraid to move forward without your partner. Do not be afraid to evolve beyond your present partner for fear of losing him/her because often the opposite is true. As one partner evolves the other frequently follows.

You may find yourself shying away from social activities you previously participated in. As you are evolving socially give yourself time to find a new way of coming together with people. Learn how to come together from a soul level. At times you may feel alone and lost between two worlds. It may seem you are growing out of one world but not quite into another. This is your spiritual adolescence. Think back to your own adolescence. You gazed upon your childhood toys, friends, and activities without interest. You longed to play with the big kids, but were not old enough. Your time will come just as it did when you were waiting to grow up. You will find a new group of friends who are spiritual adults. So do not be afraid to let go of the trappings of your spiritual youth. They will give way to glorious new experiences. Change is part of this growth process.

Have you ever noticed that when faced with change, people react quite differently? Perhaps it is important to observe, with-out judgement, how you have reacted to shifts in your life. Were you a leader? Did you move swiftly into the future excited to bring your limitless potential into full realization, energetic to see yourself and the world around you evolve and expand, or did you shrug away from the future, clinging to the past? Do you hold onto the familiar because you are afraid of the unknown? Do you deny change, ignore the signs that point to a new way of living and of doing things?

How you deal with change is crucially important at this point in time. Many opportunities are being presented to those who are able to let go of old fears, hurts, blames and consciously make a choice to move into the future. These individuals will set the tone for the future. This is a time to think in new categories. Even in the most mundane areas of your life try to think in new categories. For example, instead of fixing the same old peanut butter and jelly sandwich try adding bananas or using boysenberry jam with crushed peanuts or even pouring on chocolate syrup!

Anything goes! Get creative and move out of the same tired old way of seeing and doing things. Bring this way of being into your work, your relationships, your play time, and into your devotion. Let it breathe new life into every area of your life.

Not only will your life become much more fun but it will become much easier as well. The future is easy, the past is hard!

Our planet is being bombarded with an amazing amount of energy from our sun which increases on a daily basis. The electromagnetic activity is powerfully moving throughout this planet to help those of you who choose to be chosen utilize its energy—and move into the future. Each person must take initiative and create their own future. There are many scenarios about the future being created today. Do not buy into someone else's concept, idea or prophecy of the future. There are countless doomsday prophecies being offered. Every futuristic movie shows the Earth as a place where major disasters have destroyed most of the population. Create your own future! Remember thought directs energy. Let your thoughts come to you from a very high and clean place. Do not inherit preconceived ideas from others that resonate from a low place. As you turn a weary eye from the world of today with all its complex problems and atrocities, it is easy to see how tired you are of the way things are. Many of you are "dreamers" and know that there must be more to life than what you are currently experiencing. You long for a world filled with peace and harmony. That time is at hand. Look first to yourself. Evolve your own four natures and as you do you will see the entire planet evolving.

As I (Elizabeth), reflect on the future I recall the late John Lennon's song

"Imagine." Can you imagine a world without government, war, religion, only people living in harmony with one another, operating from a place absent of greed and malice? It's easy if you try. The future is now! The Earth has an agenda of its own and is moving into a new a direction, another dimension. It is all part of a Great Plan. The inhabitants of this beautiful globe are faced with a choice—to move forward into the future or re-main locked in the historical past. To perform God's Divine Will or to remain separated in pain and illusion. The future is never set, but continues to unfold like a flower. This is the mystery and wonder of life. The excitement is in the creative process. The choice is yours.

Let us look at a future world where there is still a birth process, a way for a soul to enter this world. Both parents would be at the birth to greet a new soul's arrival. They would rejoice at the birth of a soul that chose them as biological parents. This new soul would begin his/her life with the knowledge that s/he was wanted and celebrated, retaining the wisdom of past life lessons. The young soul would receive a balanced love from both mother and father. The apprenticeship would emphasize helping the child learn its own power as an internal force of strength, along with love, compassion and wisdom. Harmony rather than conflict would be the model for change. Evolution of self with satisfaction of accomplishments would become the primary goal. Both masculine and feminine natures would be developed equally. There would be a balance of nurturing (feminine aspect) and drive (masculine aspect).

Schools would allow students to work at their own pace and aptitude choosing their own curriculum. Such subjects could include teleportation, transcendence through the spiritual levels, of time and space travel, the nature of love, the study of the planet as a living entity, the study of this Universe and Earth's place in the cosmos, the study and integration of past philosophies into that of future philosophies. Sciences and mathematics would focus on the use of intuition and creative expression. The practice of meditation would be incorporated into every curriculum. Each child's unique gifts and talents would be nurtured and the emphasis placed on helping children uncover their divine purpose. Ways to develop the sense of intuition to its fullest extent would become the thread joining all courses. Sabbaticals for individual study would be encouraged as a tool to further instill confidence and individual creativity. Parental involvement in educative activities would be encouraged. Studies would be approached in a holistic way, emphasizing the connectedness of all things. The focus would be to help students appreciate the fact that for every physical phenomenon there exists a counterpart in the non physical realities, As above, so below. Spirituality would be integrated into every aspect of daily living, no longer seen as a separate activity but a living force in everything you do and think. Reverence for life would flow into even the most mundane of activities. The ignorance of sin, (incorrect thinking), would be dispensed through the loving education of correct thinking. Self responsibility would be the umbrella under which your apprenticeship would evolve.

Once the apprenticeship was completed, the student would begin his/her journeyman's career by moving beyond his/her parent's love and guidance out into the world. Biological parents would be seen as two loving souls who served as a way to enter this reality as well as teachers who shared many gifts and laid out the foundation of correct thinking for the newly incarnated soul. During the apprenticeship period, certain desires and interests would appear. These desires would be developed into skills and expertise. The direction of that development, career, life's purpose, is affirmed by the Universe through the individual's curiosity and drive to uncover and evolve disciplines of interest. There is a rejoicing of one's soul when an individual is given the opportunity to develop a career which aligns itself with one's life purpose. The flow of events along one's career path is the Universe's way of affirming that alignment.

If spiritual partners recognize each other along the way of their individual journeys, then a partnership is created between two souls. This partnership recognizes the need for each individual to work on his/her own story as well as the story of the partnership. Spiritual partners know that the partnership has at its core individuals, so there is respect for the needs of the individual as well as the needs for the partnership. When all four aspects of their natures are integrated into the partnership, a home becomes a source of love and nurturing.

The structure of homes could be another reflection of the harmony which exists inside you. No longer will structures require vast amounts of external energy sources to heat and cool, but will work with the available elements of the sun, wind and rain to provide comfort in your daily living. These homes will be environmentally friendly and selfsufficient. You could raise your own food in passive solar green houses, patios or vegetable gardens. Your drinking water could be collected from rain water in underground cisterns or private wells in conjunction with purification systems. Building materials would be gathered from recyclable sources. In the preparation of meals, food would be blessed with thoughts of love and nourishment for the best utility of your bodies.

Love making between two souls would be seen as a celebration of the spirit; an act of blending two energies through the sexual arousal of the Kundalini energy. If a seed is planted by the male, and the female accepts it, then another soul begins its sojourn of discovery by coexisting and cocreating with the Light.

As you progress along your journey, you eventually become a Master. As Masters you have achieved the life's lessons you came here to learn. You continue in the service of humanity in whatever capacity you are called upon by the Creator. If you are called to perform as a new breed of healers, having first become whole yourself, you will help restore balance to the afflicted in all four natures and bring him/her back to wholeness. Hospitals will also evolve their role to act as true Healing Centers playing a vital role in every society integrating all aspects of healing under one roof. As you touch larger numbers of individuals your teaching and guidance will heal those with whom you choose to share your Light. You will then move forward into the ranks of a true healer/teacher and help to midwife our planet into its magnificent future. There will be those individuals who do not choose to utilize this time frame to accelerate their spiritual evolvement. They must be permitted to move at their own pace. However, those who have not raised their vibration to a certain frequency will be unable to exist on our planet as its vibrational frequency increases.

As civilizations advance toward the new millennium, technologies will evolve in accordance with the Divine Will of the Creator. Self responsibility will be incorporated into scientific advancement. As you learn to be in complete and total harmony with God and join the Creator in the dance of creation you become a cocreator and help to give birth to a new world filled with a radiating love beyond any level you have ever before experienced. In this world human beings will work together in perfect harmony with themselves, others, Mother Earth, extraterrestrials and the Creator. You will learn how to move beyond dis- ease in all four bodies never again feeling alone, disconnected, unloved, or unworthy. You will be granted dominion over land, all the material and life everlasting. It is possible! You need to allow yourself to believe in the possibility and begin your first steps along "The Pathway Home." It is our hope that these chapters will help some of you reach the goal of Godrealization within this lifetime and learn to function from a place of higher consciousness as you move along your pathway. Remember, Home is a state of being, a level of awareness that will bring with it many, many possibilities.

SAT NAM

BIBLIOGRAPHY

Barnard, Neal, M.D. *Food for Life.* New York, N.Y.: Grown Publishers, Inc., 1993.

Chopra, Deepak, M.D. *Perfect Health.* New York, N.Y.: Crown Publishers,1991. Fortune, Dion. *The Mystical Qabalah.* York Beach, ME: Samuel Weiser, 1994. First Edition England, 1935.

Gawain, Shakti. *Living in theLight.* Novato, CA: Nataraj Publishing Co., 1986. Hesse, Hermann. *Siddhartha.* New York, NY: New Directions Publishing Corp., 1951.

Hippocrates: The Great Books of the Western World.

Vol. 20. Hippocratic Writings: University of Chicago Press, 1987. *HolyBible-King James Version.* Grand Rapids, MI: Zondervan Publishing House, 1962.

Keen, Sam, PHD. *Hymns to an Unknown God.* New York, NY: Bantam Books, 1994.

Knight, J.Z. *Ramtha.* Bellevue, WA: Sovereignty Publishers, 1986.

KublerRoss, Elisabeth, M.D. *On Death and Dying.* New York: Collier Books, McMillan Publishing Co., 1969.

Leadbeater, C.W. *The Chakras.* Wheaton, IL: The Theosophical Publishing House, 1927.

Lonsdorf, Nancy, M.D., Butler, Veronica, M.D. And Brown, Melanie, PHD. *A Woman's Best Medicine.* New York, NY: G. P. Putnam and Sons, 1993.

Monroe, Robert A. *Far Journeys* . New York, NY: Doubleday, 1985.

Monroe, Robert A. *Journeys Out of theBody.* New York, NY: Doubleday, 1971.

Monroy, Elizabeth. *TheMagical Mist.* Parker, AZ: Going Home Books, 1995.

Monroy, Elizabeth. M.S. Peter, Monroy M.D. *The Infinite Human.* Infinite Human Productions, 2022

Morningstar, Amadea., Desai, Urmila. *TheAyurvedic Cookbook.* Wilmot, WI: Lotus Press,1990. Murray, Michael T., N.D.Rocklin, CA: Prima Publishing, 1993. O'Hara, Sharon. *PearlsFrom theMoon: RaysFrom TheSun.* Bridger, MT: The Growing Place, 1994.

Ophiel. *TheArt and Practice ofAstral Projection.* York Beach, ME: Samuel Weiser, Inc., 1992.

Ornish, Dean, M.D. *Program for Reversing Heart Dis- ease.* New York, N.Y.: Ballantine Books, 1990.

Roman, Sanaya. *Spiritual Growth-Beingyour Higher Self.* Tiburon, CA: H.J. Kramer Inc., 1987.

Siegel, Bernie S., M.D. *Love, Medicine and Miracles.* New York, NY: Harper and Row, 1986.

Steere, David, PHD. *Bodily Expressions in Psychotherapy.* New York, NY :Brunner/ Mazel, 1982.

Still, William T. *New World Order.* Layfayette, Louisiana: Huntington House Publishers, 1990.

Sugrue, Thomas. *TheStory of Edgar Cayce.* Virginia Beach, VA:A.R.E. Press, 1942.

Webster's New World College Dictionary. New York, NY: Simon and Schuster and McMillan Co, 1996. f

Wilson, Ann. *Pavlov's Children.* St. Clair, Missouri: J. W. Publishing Company, 1994.

Yogananda, Paramahansa, Yogi. *Autobiography of a Yogi.* Los Angeles, CA: SelfRealization Fellowship, 1974.

Zukau, Gary. *Seat of theSoul.* New York, NY: Simon and Schuster, 1989.

FILMOGRAPHY

2001: A Space Odyssey

(1968) Alien Nation

(1988) All the President's Men

(1976) Always

(1989) The Andromeda Strain

(1971) Anna to the Infinite Power

(1984) Audrey Rose

(1977) Born Free

(1966) Brainstorm

(1983) The Cardinal

(1963) Chances Are

(1989) China Syndrome

(1979) Close Encounters of the Third Kind

(1977) Communion

(1989) CourtMartial of Billy Mitchell

(1955) Cry Freedom

(1987) The Day After,

(1983) The Day the Earth Stood Still

(1951) Dead Poets Society

(1989) The Diary of Anne Frank

(1959) The Doctor

(1991) Dr. Strangelove or How I Learned to Stop Worrying and Love the Bomb

(1964) Few Good Men

(1992) Fire in the Sky

(1993) Forbidden Planet

(1956) Gandhi

(1982) Ghost

(1990) Intruders

(1994) It's a Wonderful Life

(1946) Judgment at Nuremberg

(1961) Network

(1975) Outbreak

(1995) Paper Chase

(1973) The Philadelphia Experiment

(1984) Powder

(1995) Star Trek

(1995) Star Wars

(1977) Starman

(1984) The Secret of Santa Vittoria

(1969) You Can't Take It With You

GLOSSARY

Allopathic medicine: Modern by product of the Healing Arts which treats physical illnesses through a process of diagnosis and treatment based on cellular responses to specific pharmacological drugs or surgical removal of diseased parts.

Animalsoul: Lower aspect of the human anatomically corresponding to the old brain which is closely associated with basic survival instinctual responses.

Antioxidants: Naturally occurring chemical compounds or substances that neutralize carcinogenic free radicals particles that are consumed when eating flesh or commercially chemically laden food products.

As above, so below: Similarities which exist between the subparticle and the cosmos. What is true for the smallest unit is also true for all of Creation.

Ascended Masters: Teachers from the past, present and future who have achieved Godrealization. Some have maintained their physical bodies through transmutation to share their wisdom and knowledge with humans in the physical as well as other civilizations elsewhere in the cosmos.

Astral body: Third of five bodies the human possesses which can travel at a much faster than the speed of light. This body is usually occupied during dreams or meditative states. It remains attached to the physical body by way of a silver cord emanating from the root chakra or sacral area. This cord is severed at the death of the physical body.

Ayuverdic Medicine: Knowledge of the totality of life. Ancient holistic medicine based on the principle of body types contain ing degrees of the universal elements (air, water, fire, earth and ether) present in every individual. Nutritional diet and lifestyle counseling is then tailored to individual body type needs.

Carcinogenic substances: Any substance in foods or the environment known to cause cancer, such as free radicals.

Celestial beings: Nonspecific name given to any living entity that resides either off planet Earth in this Universe or a native from another Universe.

Chakras: Energy vortices or wheels which exist in the etheric space that coincide with strategic locations in the physical body. Their function, when activated, is to bring more of the Creator!s Light into all organs, tissues and cells rendering vitality.

Christ: Level of consciousness or office held in spiritual hierarchy.

Christ consciousness: Level of awareness reached when the consciousness is transmuted and operates from the highest spiritual plane or Sat Nam.

Cohealer: Evolved role the patient assumes with his/her healer to bring about complete wellness in all four of his/her natures acting selfresponsibly.

Dead Sea Scrolls: Eight hundred scrolls or ancient manuscripts of which only twentyfive to thirty percent have been shared with the public. Mostly written by an ascetic Jewish sect who lived in the Qumran settlement on the western shore of the Dead Sea during the time Jesus the Christ was incarnated. Many of the manuscripts were written by Jesus himself. Many of the scrolls contain references to extraterrestrial life and are now the property of the Rockefeller Museum in Jerusalem.

Ego: Personality self anatomically located at the cervical vertebrae level which filters information according to learned belief systems.

Electromagnetic being: Human physical property which maintains our physical shape working with the love force.

Energy work: The ability to effect electromagnetic changes in an individual and/or the environment to increase the vibrational frequency resulting in a faster spiritual evolution.

Etheric body: Second body the human possesses which follows the exact same contour as the physical body and extends a few millimeters to several inches in width from the physical body. This body is visible in dimly lit areas as a glowing light surrounding the physical body.

Freedome: Free head. Choosing a life path independent of social expectations.

Godrealization: Transmuted physical body and consciousness achievableonly when ground zero or karmic neutrality is reached.

Godsoul: Higher aspect of the human corresponding to the frontal cortex which is in direct contact with the Universal Mind acting as a single atom capable of limitless consciousness.

Grace: Energy descending from the creative force which if properly used by the recipient can create quantum leaps in that soul!s spiritual evolution. Those who receive this gift from God must humble and soften themselves in order to properly receive it.

Healer: Evolved member of the Healing Arts who integrates the patient's four natures in his/her treatment protocol.

HealingArts: The Science of allowing Divine Principle to flow through the physical body by treating physical, emotional, mental and spiritual dis- eases to bring about total wholeness.

Herbal cleansing: Use of medicinal herbs for the purpose of detoxifying various organs in the body.

Herbology: Medical science which deals with the use of herbs for medicinal purposes.

Higher self: Spiritual body which everyone possesses that functions with greater awareness than the physical body and connects to the higher spiritual planes working as an intermediator between the ego and the soul.

Hippocrates: Father of modern medicine born in the Island of Kos, Greece (400 BG) and founder of holistic medicine.

Homeopathic Medicine: Medical science which deals with the use of homeopathic remedies.

Homeopathic remedies: Treatment of dis- eases based on the administration of minute doses of a drug (usually an herb) that in massive doses produces symptoms in healthy individuals similar to those of the dis- ease itself.

Kundalini: In Sanskrit meaning the serpent power which lies dormant in the root chakra anatomically corresponding to the gonadal area. Arousal of this powerful divine energy through meditation, sexual intercourse or spontaneously can lead to heightened levels of consciousness or mental illness in the event the subject is unprepared.

Law of Karma: Universal law of Cause and Effect.

Levitation: Ability to transcend gravitational forces and float in mid air seen in some individuals during deep meditative states who are close to achieving Christ consciousness.

Light body: Transmuted body which operates from Sat Nam.

Macrocosm: The cosmos.

Management: A hierarchy of evolved entities assigned to over see and carry out the Divine Will of God. Management works with every carnated soul to orchestrate life experiences to maximize the individual!s spiritual journey. The usual mode of communication is through the sense of intuition and physical signs placed synchronistically along that soul!s pathway.

Microcosm: The human.

Nutritional Medicine: Medical science which deals with diet and proper absorption of physical nourishment.

Pavlov's dogs: Russian physiologist who described conditioned behavioral responses in dogs based on a system of punishment and rewards depending on their behavior.

Physical body: Composite of four bodies (physical, emotional, mental and spiritual) which represents a holy temple granted to the carnating soul to complete karmic debts and/or carry out the Creator!s Will on this planet.

Preventive lifestyle: Developing the awareness that a lifetime represents a series of opportunities given the individual to complete karmic lessons. This higher sense of purpose includes the acceptance of the physical body as a living temple which implies a nurturing physical, emotional, mental and spiritual diet.

Purpose: Life agenda prepared prior to incarnating with the assistance of management. The duty of each soul to carry out the Creator!s Divine Will through their own creative and unique actions.

Reincarnation: Process by which a soul!s life energy is slowed down by its attraction to the gravitational forces of a planet that requires payment of karmic debts through actions in the physical plane. The recycling process through birthdeath continues (Wheel of Karma) until all debts are repaid, at that point the entity assumes its natural spiritual state and is given the opportunity to exist in spirit or form unattached to any specific planet and for all eternity.

Sat Nam: First Plane of manifestation, fifth or soul level which translates in Sanskrit to mean "Truth be Its Name."

Skinner!s pigeons: Famous American psychologist!s experiment dealing with stimulus-response behavior in trained pigeons.

Synapse: Junction point through which sensory information is transmitted to various parts of the physical body.

Synchronicity: Series of similar events which to the unaware soul could be misconstrued as coincidence. These events are symbolized messages from management to the individual, which if properly interpreted, can hasten the individual!s complete soul unfoldment.

Teleportation: Ability to dematerialize physical body and travel through the ethers and rematerialize in another location.

The Great Plan: All manifestations are part of a single Creator's expired breath which lasts approximately 26,000 Earth years. At the next inspiration cycle, which lasts another 26,000 years, all accumulated knowledge from the cosmos is then returned to the Creator to start a new breathing cycle. The ultimate purpose of all manifestations is to increase the Creator!s knowledge through the actions of all living things.

Third party payers: Any organization, insurance company or government which pays for medical services.

Thought form: Energy pattern or vortex that exists in the ethers and is created by an individual or group soul which can affect the consciousness of those who come in contact with it in a positive or negative manner.

Toxins: Substances which are known to be harmful to the physical body usually derived from man's cancerous behavior with his host, the planet Earth.

Transmutation: Process by which a third of the cells are detoxified from the physical body through correct physical, emotional, mental and spiritual actions as well as special natural agents, which then allows the individual to receive more of the Creator!s Light instantly transmuting every cell by resonating at a higher frequency. This holy act always takes place after the individual!s consciousness has reached Godrealization. The physical body is always transmuted in front of witnesses and is accompanied by the sound of music.

Universal Mind: Super consciousness which exists at the lower regions of the mental plane and is accessible through the sense of intuition and meditation. Anyone who can gain access is able to extract information from this limitless source.

Universe: Plane of existence which encompasses all of creation in a particular electromagnetic frequency range. There are at least 91,000 to the 91th power Universes. The physical Universe represents a single cell in cosmic terms.

Yinyang: Passive, female principle constantly interacting with the male, active principle to bring harmony in all living things.

Yogi: A person who seeks union with God.

A

Acupuncture 12

As above so below 182.190

Ascended Masters 190.19, 175, 5, 122,

Animalsoul 190

Antioxidants 190 Astral 59,61,187,190

Aura 36, 117 Ayruvedic 12

B

Babaji 122

Bible 89, 112, 116118, 121,164 Buddha 50, 110,119, 122123

C

Christians 119,122 Cofacilitators 7

Co-healer 3,8,15 Caudeus 17

Chakra 16,84,126,190, 192 Chakras 16,50,66,114, 186.191 Cardinal Humors 6

Chiropratics 12

Christ 5051, 110,

114115,119,122,191, 193

Christian 68,118120,

122,127 133,137,153,163,178 146148, 150

D

Detoxification 83 Detoxified 194 Detoxifying 192 Diaphragmatic 26

Dis- ease 78, 1214, 17, 2830,35,4041, 6465, 67, 69, 71,144

Dis- eased 1,3,10,64

E

Educate 17, 30, 35,100, 130, 168 Educated 147

Educating 143

Educational 142, 144,

Egos 7,13

Egotistical 70

Einstein 19,58 Electrochemical 8, 24, 35

Electrochemically 46

Electromagnetic 17, 19, 26,

113114,181,191,195

Emotion 20, 30, 40,162

Emotionally 32, 37, 47, 76, 9697,105,129131,

Emotionless 155 Empowerment 83 Energy 181 Enlightened 17 Enlightment 169

Environment 2, 6, 17, 25,

65, 68, 72,79, 83, 165, 190191

Environmental 17,145 Equanimity 34, 37, 95, 160 Ethe r 190 Etheric 114, 191

Extraterrestrials 117

F

Foundation

109, 131,147, 149, 160, 183

13, 29, 65, 97, Foundations 148

G

Gods 5,117

God 62,152,174 Godaspect 56

Godrealization 50,100, 120, 123, 137138, 160, 185,190,192,195

Godsoul 192

Governments 73,119 Greedily 105 Governmental 113, 123 81, 99, 101 Greedy 76,

89

H

Heirachy 140

Herbology 2, 12, 192

Herbs 25, 192

Hippocrates 2, 6, 186, 192

Hippocratic 2, 9, 186

Holistic 6,14, 70, 89, 182, 190,192

Holy 3, 16, 66, 84, 108, 110, 115, 117, 131, 137, 156,186,193194

Home 4, 6, 810,12, 14, 16, 20, 2224, 2628, 32, 34, 36, 38, 4244,4648,5051,54,56, 58, 60, 62, 66, 68, 70, 72, 74, 76, 78, 80, 82, 84, 86, 90, 92, 94, 96, 98, 100, 102, 104106, 110, 112114, 116, 118, 120,122123, 126128, 130132, 134, 136, 138, 140, 142, 144, 146, 148, 150,152,154,156, 158159,162, 164166, 168, 170174, 176186, ; 188, 190, 192, 194, 196, 198, 200, 202, 204, 206, 208, 210, 212, 214, 216, 218, 220, 222, 224

I

Imagination 150,154

Incarnate 50 2, 192 57, 101, 128, 103104

Incarnated 112113,122, 150,183,191 Incarnating 19, 42,119, 138, 193

Intuition 5, 1012, 26, 36, 45, 72, 95,104, 111, 126, 147148, 168, 176, 182,193,195

J

Jesus
114115,122, 169,191

K

Karma
56, 6162, 67, 88,101, 111113,119,121, 166167, 193

Karmic 4,13, 23, 32, 50, 61, 67,101,112113, 116,120,172,192193

Karmically 14, 23, 105

Kundalini 1617,114,131, 184.192 Light body 51,114,193 Lovemaking 44, 126, 130131

Lucid 48-49 M

5, 50, 56,110,

Mantrum 156, 179

Matrix 57, 111

Maya 33, 62

Medicaid 9,73 77,79, 81 83, 85 Medicare 9, 73, 75 77, 79, 81 83, 85, 94 13, 23, 32, 38, 50,

L

Laparoscopic Laparoscopy Levitation 114, 193 Meditations 24

Meditative 63,190, 193

Mentally 27,41,47,76, 96 97,130 131,137, 153,163,178 Microcosm 19 20, 175, 193 Mindbody dis- ease 30

Lifestyle 2, 6, 89, 14 15, 77, 83, 95,163, 174, 190.193

Light 33, 39, 50 51, 55, 58, 66, 72, 83, 85,107,114, 119,121,130,160, 177 178,184,186, 190 191,193 194

O

Out of body 114 57, 59 60,

74, 83 11, 85 Muhammad

N

Neurotransmitters 35 Nirvana 34 Macrocosm 193

19 20,175,

Meditate Meditating Meditation 56, 59, 63,179 o, 111 27, 59 60, 108, 115,156,182,192,195 122 123

P

Parent 36, 46, 68 69, 75, 84,103,133 135,148, 150,153 154,163,183

Parental 182

Parenthood 131

Parenting 103, 131, 133 Playful 46,151

Playfulness 151,154 156 Prana 26, 56, 66

Prayer 23,108,115, 156 157 Prayers 157

Praying 111,121

Prophecies 181

Prophecy 181

Prophetic 167

Psychiatrists 70

Psychiatry 16

Psychic 109

Psychological 68,148

Psychologist 194

Psychologists 70

Psychology 16

Psychotherapist 162

Psychotherapists 31

Psychotherapy 187

Purification 21, 49, 52, 72, 83,172,183 Purified i21,' 68 Purify 21 Purifying 121

R

Rajdiance 67

Radiate 43

Radiates 5, 66 Radiating 66, 178, 184 Radiation 178

Recreate 42

Reincarnate 61

Reincarnation 112, 121, 193 Religioeducative 17

Religions 61,110, 114, 118, 121, 160

Religiopolitical Reprogram 46 Reprogrammed 127 Rhythm 25,69,169 Rockefeller 148,191

Root 16, 71, 126,190,192 Roswell 169

Rothschild 148 s

S

Sat Nam 62,156,185,191, 193194 Science 2, 6, 24,116,148, 162,192193 Scientific 184

2, 7, 182,1011, 65, 116,

Scientifically 116 Scientist 116

Scientists 26, 58,117 Self love 21 114., 118

Selfrealized 40

Selfgoverning 98, 107

Selfgovernment 105

Symbolizes 98,107,112, 125126,150 Symbolizing 17, 56, 134

Symbols 49,52,169,176

Synapse 4647, 194

Separate 112, 164, 171, 182

Separated 75, 116, 181

Separateness 16, 32, 56, 72, 99, 112

Separates 6

Separating 66, 106 2, 25, 59, 65, 91, 127, 134, 138, 162,

Synapses 4546

Separation 1516, 59, 66, 72, 112, 128 Synchronicity 155,168, 194 Synchronistically 193 Sex 34, 89, 125, 128129, 131,133,136137,142 Sexes 128129

Sexual 4, 42, 49, 130131, 184,192

Sexuality 130 Sexually 161 Siddhartha 186 Spacecraft 117 Spaceship 165

Spirituality 0; 3, 16, 28, 54, 56, 62, 88,106,116, 118, 161,171, 182

Stars 117, 173

Symbol 17,131,177

Symbolic 48, 52, 68, 97, 108,170

Symbolically 175 Symbolize 19, 23, 56 Symbolized 60,174, 194

5, 7778, 119

T

Teach 13,114,121,132, 137,146,148,154

Teacher 6, 13, 62, 94, 114, 118,139, 144145,150, 184

Teaches

Teaching 166167, 184

Teachings 2, 61,109, 111, 114115 Teleportation 114,182,194

Temple 20, 56, 8384,110, 131.160.165.193 Temples 126, 132

Therapies 83

Therapist 31, 137 Therapists 162 Therapy 12,14 Transcendence 182 Transcending

116, 151

Transcends 61,128

Transmutation 5051, 59, 114.177,190.194,148, 150, Transmute 116

Transmuted 50, 191193

Transmuting 17, 194

V

Vegetarian 2325, 27, 60 Vegetarians 23 Veggie 24

Vibrant 148

Vibrates 50

Vibration 19, 6162, 116, 130, 178, 184 Vibrational 30, 32, 40, 51, 113, 184, 191

W

Wheels 4,117

Y

Yinyang 53, 195 Yogananda 187 Yogi 187,195

www.ingramcontent.com/pod-product-compliance
Lightning Source LLC
Chambersburg PA
CBHW020248010526
44107CB00002B/150